Communication Skills that Heal

A practical approach to a new professionalism in medicine

Barry Bub MD

Radcliffe Publishing
Oxford • Seattle

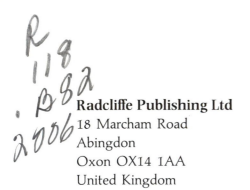

Radcliffe Publishing Ltd
18 Marcham Road
Abingdon
Oxon OX14 1AA
United Kingdom

www.radcliffe-oxford.com
Electronic catalogue and worldwide online ordering facility.

British Library Cataloguing in Publication Data

A catalogue record for this book is available from the British Library.

ISBN-10: 1 85775 664 9
ISBN-13: 978 1 85775 664 7

Typeset by Aarontype Ltd, Easton, Bristol
Printed and bound by TJ International Ltd, Padstow, Cornwall

For Goldie

Contents

Frontispiece

Meaning is not a fixity. It does not exist encoded in the words of any single book. It is a function of the dynamic interaction between the reader and the read, at the contact/boundary itself. Meaning is the ever-shifting, infinitely various figure that emerges from the destructuring of what is read, what is heard, or what is observed — what is experienced. Without this destructuring, 'meaning' would remain an alien introject, dead clumps of authority exerting a leaden weight on the liveliness of true understanding.

Dan Bloom, *Song of the Self*, November 1993

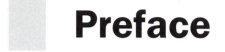

Preface

> We have two ears and one mouth
> so we may listen more and talk the less.
> Epictetus, 55 AD–135 AD[1]

The ritual

'Good! Now we can sit in one large circle and face each other.' Satisfied that I had rearranged the furniture satisfactorily, I returned to silently rehearsing my speech.

The examination room had been changed in many other ways. The desktop was now bare. Gone were photos of wife, children, and grandchildren, little mementos from travels, Post-It notes, and pens. The cabinet counters too had been cleared of their paraphernalia. Tongue depressors, alcohol swabs, cotton balls, Band-Aids, and syringes were now hibernating in boxes on the floor. This was a room in transition, stripped down to its essentials, and waiting for the movers.

Some hints of the ambience carefully crafted over the years remained however. Classical music drifted over the intercom. A cut-glass vase filled with roses and lilies from the front garden rested on an end table. Framed photographs (24 × 36 inches) of idyllic nature scenes still hung on the eggshell-white walls. Long-since gone were glossy wall charts of narrowed coronary arteries, smokers' black lungs, and fungating colon cancers that were gifts from pharmaceutical companies, since this was an environment designed to calm rather than educate or intimidate apprehensive patients.

Now, what remained of this ambience was sorely needed to soothe my frazzled nerves.

It had been a very difficult day. All afternoon a lump had been massaging my throat as I said my final goodbyes to patients. I had been anticipating and dreading this day for weeks. Grief welled up at the mere thought of seeing the appointment book blank and the filing cabinet emptied of charts for the coming week. This would be no mere vacation. When I left the office, it would be never to return.

I had been practicing solo family medicine here since 1975, and even though my practice had been financially rewarding, the impeding healthcare and litigation crises in Pennsylvania made it imperative that we physicians take collective action if disaster was to be averted. Despite my involvement in organized medicine, I could not shake my colleagues in our medical community from their collective apathy. There was little future for solo medicine, so I eventually sold my practice to a regional hospital network, receiving a lucrative contract to work as a physician employee. A major attraction was their promise of professional management and a stable supportive network, neither of which materialized. Three years later, with patient safety being threatened by corporate policies, I quietly informed my patients of my impending departure. Now, on the eve of a potentially disastrous merger with another practice, we were to have our closing ritual.

This entire period was very distressing. Fortunately, a few weeks earlier, some friends and I had brainstormed what would be needed to make this awesome transition less painful and more meaningful. We decided that a ritual was called for. A ritual would enable me to leave the office, not alone, but with support. It would also acknowledge that the work we had done in the office had been special, even perhaps, as my wife suggested, 'holy'. Rather than simply vacate the building to its next occupant, a ritual would allow us to *deconsecrate* the space, and say goodbye.

Monica, our perennially cheerful receptionist, was the first to enter the room. She startled me with her reddened eyes and box of tissues clutched firmly in her hand. 'What's this?' I wondered. Immersed in my own sorrow, and thinking that this was just another job for my employees, it just hadn't occurred to me that they would be particularly distressed. 'Who is giving support to whom today?' I wondered.

Terry and Liz entered the room. Their exuberant cheerfulness seemed forced rather than real. Donna, our office assistant, on the other hand appeared subdued. Anna and her husband John, long-time patients, arrived bearing gifts, and took their seats in the circle. One empty seat remained. Joan, our nurse, who was normally so unflappable, seemed to be taking longer than usual cleaning up at the end of the day. 'Is she procrastinating, apprehensive at the prospect of this closing ceremony?' I went to find her.

Finally we were all seated. Chatter settled down. Even though the ritual had barely begun, I noticed that there was already a perceptible shift of energy. No longer a hierarchy, we were now just a small group of people joined together in marking a transition. Now my carefully rehearsed speech seemed contrived and inappropriate, so I set it aside, leaned back, and listened.

Terry, our office manager, spoke of the time I had fired her for insubordination (unfairly, she thought), only to visit her in hospital a few months later after she had been injured in a serious automobile accident. She eventually returned to our practice, becoming a model employee and later manager. She wept as she told how much this had meant to her.

Joan recalled the day she was hired, terrified, having heard how demanding I could be. Then, as she gained experience, she learned to value herself and the work she did, often insisting with pride as she compared us with others, 'This is *NOT* the way it's done at Dr Bub's!'

The others each took their turn, all except John who was mildly demented. He just smiled, seemingly enjoying the experience.

Finally, it was time for me to speak. By now, I was feeling very humbled and moved. I allowed the words to spill out.

'We have had many office meetings over the years,' I began, 'and this is the first one that started off by me listening to *you*. How different would my life have been had I begun my career by listening rather than speaking? What if medical practice had included *listening* practice?'

They smiled at this, but for me these were more than trite questions. I thought of stressed and dissatisfied employees quitting unexpectedly; long-time patients leaving the practice for no apparent reason; my own divorce. How much hardship had been caused or aggravated by my inability to listen?

Sadness turned to indignation as I realized that I had been as much victim as perpetrator. It had not all been my fault; the culture of medicine just did not encourage listening. 'I trusted my teachers and the leaders of my profession to focus on the important,' I pointed out, 'yet I don't recall ever being to a medical lecture or conference where the topic was listening.' Two encounters came to mind as I spoke – the first at the beginning of my career, and the second almost 30 years later, as I was to transition to another phase.

The hyperventilator

'It frightens me, Doctor. I have these spells where I can't get enough air so I breathe fast. My head becomes dizzy, and my fingers fall asleep.' With a waiting room full of patients, there was too little time to have this middle-aged lady disrobe. A perfunctory examination through her thin cotton dress was unremarkable. Besides, the history was classic, and as a newly minted medical graduate, I was excited at having diagnosed my first case of hyperventilation syndrome.

'No need to worry, your symptoms can all be explained by anxiety. You'll be fine,' I reassured her. After advising her how to abort these episodes, I suggested she return for a complete physical. Then I walked her to the door.

At the threshold of the doorway, with one foot outside the room, in a typical *fight or flight* or *hand on the doorknob* position, she turned to face me and asked, 'May I show you something?' I nodded. Shutting the door behind her, she dropped one shoulder strap of her flimsy dress, and undid her bra. Her right breast had been replaced by an enormous fungating cancer — something she had earlier been too terrified to reveal.

In my excitement at making my diagnosis, I had not thought to ask an obvious question: '*Why* are you feeling so anxious?'

Listening had just not been on my agenda.

The psychiatrist

Just a few weeks before our closing ritual, I joined 19 other primary care physicians in a teleconference on the topic of depression. The case of a 40-year-old woman with anxiety and depression was the vehicle for a seemingly endless journey into the minutiae of the latest 'me too' antidepressant.

Increasingly uncomfortable with this approach, I asked the psychiatrist discussion leader, 'What if the patient is anxious and depressed because her husband is abusing her and lives in an unhealthy and possibly dangerous environment? Maybe she needs less medication and more listening?'

There was silence on the phone, then the 'expert' stammered, 'Oh yes, of course ... always take a history.' He hastily thanked us and ended the session before we could pursue this uncomfortable line of discussion any further.

'No, not much had changed in 30 years,' I told our little circle of ritual participants.

We concluded our ritual walking from room to room, symbolically taking down photographs from walls, distributing them, and then turning off the lights. Finally, we went outside and unscrewed the nameplate:

BARRY BUB M.D.
FAMILY PRACTICE

Many hugs, shared gifts, and a few tears later, we adjourned as a group to a restaurant where we celebrated with food, wine, and fond memories of favorite patients.

Like an acrobat, I had let go of the trapeze ...

Barry Bub
July 2005

Reference

1   www.quotationspage.com/quotes/Epictetus (accessed 27 June 2005).

About the author

Always a creative, independent thinker, Barry Bub has frequently applied non-conventional solutions to professional challenges. As a medical student, he found pediatric lectures muddled, and he ignored them, choosing instead to create his own system of independent study. The result: Barry was the first person in the history of the university to win all the pediatric prizes.

Following cum laude graduation from the University of Cape Town at the tender age of 22, and wanting to practice holistic medicine, he resisted offers of specialization, and elected instead to pursue a career in family medicine.

Four years later, he emigrated from apartheid-era South Africa to the USA, where he applied principles of *Total Quality Improvement* and *Time Expansion* to develop a highly successful family practice.

A 32-hour work week provided him the freedom to: teach at a residency program; study graphoanalysis, useful for rapidly assessing patients' psychological status; complete a 3-year training program in Gestalt psychotherapy to improve relationship and counseling skills; and assume a leadership role in organized medicine via presidencies of the hospital medical staff and various medical organizations.

Following his departure from active medical practice, he moved to Manhattan where he joined the New York Gestalt Institute, practiced psychotherapy, taught counseling skills to clergy, entered a chaplaincy training program and studied Focusing and personality disorders. Following the September 11th terror attack, he worked as a volunteer chaplain for the American Red Cross. This kindled his interest in the role of trauma in medicine and the role of communication in healing.

Dr Bub now innovates novel teaching concepts from various disciplines such as chaplaincy and psychotherapy; lectures and leads creative interactive workshops for healthcare professionals on topics related to communication, counseling and self-care. He confidentially counsels healthcare professionals and clergy who are experiencing litigation and professional stress. He is author of several journal articles and the website www.processmedicine.com. He is a member of the AMA/CMA committee that plans an international conference on physician health. He is also a regular presenter at medical schools, hospitals and national medical conferences and meetings.

Barry Bub is married, the proud father of three children and grandfather of six.

Acknowledgements

It was a glorious spring day, a day for hiking a mountain or sitting on a park bench in a sunbeam. Yet there I was, indoors and hard at work editing this book. 'What internalized taskmaster compels me to do this?' I asked myself.

The answer was simply that the University of Cape Town Medical School had left me with a legacy. There I had encountered professors of enormous stature such as Stuart Saunders, Frankie Forman, Golda Seltzer, Raymond Hoffenberg, Ralph Ger, Arderne Forder, Helen Brown, Lennox Eales, Jannie Louw, Velva Schrire, Hymie Gordon, and others. These were heroic figures created in the mould of Sir William Osler and they imprinted on their students an indelible image of medicine as an honorable and privileged profession. Their passion and commitment had lit a torch of humanistic professionalism which needs to be kept lit.

I have been fortunate. These great teachers and mentors have been followed by others. I think of Mark Putnam MD who encouraged me to undertake Gestalt training. He and his gifted co-teachers at the Pennsylvania Gestalt Center, Mariah Fenton Gladis MSS and Dori Middleman MD created one transformative experience after another, ever expanding my awareness in the process.

Ed Grab, formerly of the Healthcare Group, is a master of practice management and total quality improvement. His input was essential in my learning to create a solid foundation for healthy communication.

More recently, Dan Bloom, former President of the New York Gestalt Institute, has been my principal teacher of Gestalt theory, Elinor Greenberg PhD of the Masterson Institute was my teacher in personality disorders and Rabbi Bonita Taylor of the Healthcare Chaplaincy was my dedicated supervisor in chaplaincy. Eugene Gendlin PhD, the originator of Focusing, personally assigned a teacher, Bridgette Domas, to teach me this technique.

Roger Brown of the AMA nourished my interest in physician health by including me in the AMA/CMA international conference planning committee. Rabbi Dr Zalman Schachter-Shalomi entrusted me with the task of creating a Guild of medical, healthcare, and healing professionals, which is becoming a source of numerous inspiring, enriching connections.

Writing can be a very lonely experience but not with a writers' group that includes such eclectic and colorful characters as Debbie Wong, Robin

Greenstein, Paul Morrissey, and Ken Paprocki and creative non-fiction writing teacher, Michael Kaye.

Appreciation to my wife, Rabbi Goldie Milgram, for her conceptual, artistic and detail-oriented contributions to this manuscript process. Finally, thank you to my family for providing the love, caring, and support that every healthcare professional needs to do his or her work in the world.

Introduction

Anger at both ends of the stethoscope
New York Times[1]

From a physician client's files:

10/28/04

Dear Doctor,

Enclosed is a check for the balance due for my office visits last month. You may remember that I complained of chest pain. Eventually you reassured me that my heart was normal. Actually, I was not worried about my heart — you were. All I wanted was for the pain to go away. Eventually, it did, when I discovered the real cause and left my husband!

   I need you to know that when I was at your office I felt totally invisible as a person. Even though there was so much on my chest that I needed to share, all you seemed to be interested in was heart disease. If you had just inquired and listened, perhaps we could have avoided all those expensive tests. So, in addition to the check, for the sake of future patients, I would like to offer you one piece of advice.

   Drop that stethoscope and listen!

Sincerely,
Marianne Smith

11/5/04

Dear Mrs Smith,

I took a 10-minute break for lunch today, and while eating a sandwich thought I would read my mail. When I saw your letter, in its hand-addressed envelope, I was at first delighted thinking it was a thank-you note from a grateful patient. Needless to say, I almost choked when I read its contents.

Perhaps you don't appreciate that we physicians hardly have time to breathe, let alone spend time talking to our patients. Managed care requires that I see on average four patients an hour. Then I have to document the visits in detail, review lab reports, return phone calls, catch up on my journals, attend meetings, and deal with practice issues. The list is endless. How would you suggest I find the time to listen?

I consider myself a very competent physician. There have been many reports recently on cases of coronary artery disease in women that are misdiagnosed as stress and I needed to be sure that I did not make that mistake.

I'm very sorry you didn't feel heard and understood, but it could not be helped. I am not a therapist.

Feel free to transfer your records to another physician of your choice.

Sincerely,
Robert E. Jones MD

Phew! Notice how each is left hurting, traumatized and bruised. There is no place of meeting, certainly no healing, and this mirrors the world at large where patients frequently complain that physicians do not listen to and understand them,[2] and physicians in turn respond that they do not have enough time.[3] Both groups have a point.

Patients experience widespread frustration, disillusionment, cynicism, and anger.[1] When an error or perceived error occurs, this anger is frequently channeled into litigation.[4]

Physicians experience stress, negative feedback, and absence of meaning, joy, and satisfaction. High income alone does not compensate for this so well-being suffers and burnout increases.[5]

The healthcare system is stuck with escalating costs, resulting from medical mistakes, high insurance, litigation, defensive medicine, unnecessary investigations, excessive medication, and repeat visits to practitioners.

In other words, a total lose–lose situation except for some members of the legal profession.

It is terrifying being ill or having a relative who is seriously ill particularly when experienced within an increasingly impersonal healthcare system, and it is the rare individual who has not been alienated or angered by at least one seemingly insensitive, distant, or non-empathetic healthcare professional who has made matters worse by his or her style of communication. Like Marianne Smith, some individuals complain and write angry letters, and, not surprisingly, physicians who receive more complaints are at significantly higher risk of being sued.[6]

On hearing the title of this book, people invariably light up. They say, 'This is so needed', or 'Let me tell you about my experience', and then follow up with comments such as these:

- 'I wish my doctor would join the human race.'
- 'He's a wonderful doctor, but much too busy to listen.'
- 'She is excellent, but you know, her bedside manner could do with some improvement.'
- 'Thank goodness for his receptionist. Now *she* is someone I can talk to!'
- 'He writes on his laptop while I'm speaking to him. Can you imagine that? He doesn't even look at me!'
- 'As soon as I started to cry, he ran off to fetch his nurse. Don't you know doctors flee from suffering?'
- 'I was diagnosed with MS at 24 after I had suddenly lost my eyesight. He said there was no treatment for MS and that I should go and live my life. That was 9 years ago, and I can see just fine. Why could he not have offered just a little hope?'
- 'I much prefer his nurse practitioner.'
- 'I don't even bother to talk to her anymore, she never listens anyway.'
- 'He sodomized my son. Could he not have spoken to him first before shoving that sigmoidoscope up his rectum?'
- 'I feel invisible, just a cog in the medical system.'
- 'I rehearse what I'm going to say, then ask him not to interrupt me if I promise not to talk for longer than a minute.'
- 'I blessed him to have a better day. You know he never ignored me again.'
- 'I had to be really creative to get her attention, so at my prenatal visit when she breezed into the examination room and lifted my gown to expose my abdomen, she was startled to see a note taped to my protruding belly with an arrow pointing to my head. In it I had written: *Doctor, will you for once listen to me?'*

Many words have been written about the anguish of physicians[7] – as have been written about the suffering of patients[8] and their loved ones.[9] Clearly there is trauma at each end of the stethoscope. The question is whether this tug of war can be satisfactorily resolved.

I believe it can, once it is accepted that:

- both populations are suffering
- physicians and other healthcare professionals cannot fully listen, understand, empathize, and support when they themselves are traumatized, dispirited and disillusioned
- patient and professional healing and well-being are interdependent; income cannot substitute for the absence of positive feedback, meaning

and satisfaction derived from patients who feel well cared for; no one group can thrive at the expense of the other.

Rather than the downward spiral of a lose–lose relationship, what is needed is an upward spiral of healing based on skilled professional communication that facilitates healing and well-being in both patient and practitioner.

This is conditional upon the following:

- The word *healing* has to be reclaimed into general medicine to be used specifically in the context of restoration of healthy function of the individual following the physical, psychological and spiritual trauma inflicted by illness and accidents.
- For healing to improve quality of care, healing must be used to support excellent treatment rather than be a substitute for it.
- Healing needs to be appreciated as something that is never one-sided, and that both professionals and patients derive benefit in the process of healing work.
- Since healing emerges from healing relationships, medical care needs to be *relationship-centered*, not patient-centered, practitioner-centered nor disease-centered.
- For communication to heal it needs to be *authentic*, i.e., it needs to emerge from the authentic self. This form of communication is by definition highly personal since *how you listen* and *what you say* emerges from *you*, and not from lifeless parroting of scripted information. Nor is it based on acting, as suggested in a recent article, 'Clinical empathy as emotional labor in the patient–physician relationship.'[10] Here, the authors, while acknowledging that 'the healing relationship between physicians and patients remains essential to quality care', propose that practitioners engage in 'deep acting' to demonstrate empathy in a manner similar to other service workers, such as flight attendants and bill collectors.
- Authentic communication does not imply that it is unfiltered, un-processed, or uninformed by professionalism.
- Communication that is derived from a skilled and authentic self requires that the self be healthy. Unlike other medical skill-sets, with relationship skills, *what you are* is as important as *what you do*. This requires much more than the acquisition of a communication competency. It is no mere cosmetic makeover.
- Transformation of the self – whether as an individual or an institution – is far from easy. Deep down the hapless and chastised Dr Jones knows he has to improve his communication style. He is highly intelligent, yet his cleaning person is a far better listener. His colleagues acknowledge that their communication skills are inadequate.[11] His organizations and teaching institutions are aware of the problem:

Communication is a core clinical skill. In the course of a career spanning 40 years, a hospital doctor is likely to do around 150 000 to 200 000 interviews with patients and their families. However, very few doctors have received much formal training in communication, and the training provided is commonly inadequate. Senior doctors recognize that their deficiencies in this area contribute to high psychological morbidity, emotional burnout, depersonalization, and low personal accomplishments.[12]

● There needs to be a deep appreciation for the role resistance plays in slowing and limiting change. The reasons for resistance include the following.

1   Change cannot be accomplished in oneself or one's profession through *will* alone.

The truth is that fundamental change of one's self or one's professional institutions is remarkably difficult. It requires more than determination. It is basic human nature to resist change with preference given to holding onto what is familiar and feels safe hence all those self-help books that benefit their authors more than their readers.

John O Stevens, in his book *Awareness: Exploring, Experimenting, Experiencing*, makes this point:

> There are a lot of self-improvement books that tell you how to change yourself. When you try to change, you manipulate and torture yourself, and mostly you just become divided between a part of you that tries to change and a part of you that resists change. Even when you do accomplish change in this way, the price is conflict, confusion and uncertainty. Usually, the more you try to change, the worse your situation becomes.[13]

In his book *The Doctor and the Soul*, Viktor Frankl writes of the three human strivings: the will to pleasure, the will to power, and the will to meaning.[14] Will is important to the human spirit, but there are limits to the ability of will to create change in the self. Gerald G May, in his book *Will and Spirit*, points out, '... we think we should be able to control and manipulate our psyches ...' and '... the human mind has become objectified as a thing to be fixed, altered, streamlined.'[15]

Physicians mostly focus on will in an attempt to change the behavior of patients using the following formula:

- indicate the problem
- warn of the consequences if behavior does not change
- prescribe medication, diet, exercise program, quit smoking program, etc.

Inevitably little, if any, change takes place.[16] Similarly, as physicians, our prescriptions for our own behavioral changes usually fail.

There are at least two other reasons why we physicians tend not to learn communication skills that are so readily available to other professionals:

2   The biomedical model narrows options.
Robbie Davis-Floyd, a cultural/medical anthropologist, proposes that after all the years of training physicians' neural pathways are established in terms of what she calls 'the technocratic model of medicine.' Because physicians are so busy, it takes too much energy to assimilate information from outside the technocratic paradigm. New ways of thinking require the creation of new neural pathways, not easy for those under stress and just trying to cope.[17]

3   Fixed ideas first need to be critically examined and, if necessary, deconstructed.
Resistances (in Gestalt terminology) can be viewed as deep-seated beliefs that become the norms and fixities of our thinking. These *resistances* inhibit our ability to take useful action. Change in self can be accomplished through raising awareness of these *resistances*, preferably in a healing relationship within an environment of safety. People tend not to make needed changes when they feel threatened, judged, or shamed. John O Stevens articulates the issue of awareness and resistance as follows:

> ... it is much more useful to simply become deeply aware of yourself as you are now. Rather than try to change, stop, or avoid something that you don't like in yourself, it is much more effective to stay with it and become more deeply aware of it. When you really get in touch with your own experiencing, you will find that change takes place by itself, without your effort or planning. With full awareness you can let it happen with confidence that it will work out well. You can learn to let go and live and flow with your experiencing and happening instead of frustrating yourself with demands to be different. All the energy that is locked up in the battle between trying to change and resisting change can become available for participation in the happening of your life.[13]

For these reasons, acquiring communication skills requires more than the study of communication as a competency.

About this book

By now you will probably realize that this book is by no means intended to be a comprehensive manual on the subject of communication. Nor is it designed to simplify communication into a simple skill set created by someone else containing a collection of mnemonics, lists of *dos and don'ts*, or principles of communication reduced to a series of sound bites.

When communication is a purely intellectual exercise derived from memorized principles, it is flat, stiff and lacks spontaneity. When derived from a deep authentic place of self, the speaker is 'in the flow' and may even be astonished at hearing the words as they emerge, thinking, 'Wow that sounds really right. Where did these words come from?' This is a deeply satisfying and even profound experience.

What this book hopefully will do is to raise your awareness, and stimulate, provoke, and offer alternative perspectives that will lead you to communicate differently with your patients. It requires of you a commitment to your own spiritual and emotional health and well-being, with the understanding that successful communication with others will add to your personal feeling of well-being. In other words a win–win situation.

Since resistance is such a major challenge to change, the initial chapters of this book focus on uncovering and challenging the many myths and fixed images about communication and healing that you may have unconsciously assimilated in the course of your training. Each chapter then concludes with practice pointers. As old ways of behavior are unlearned, new ways are proposed. Additionally, as your awareness is raised about issues such as shame, boundaries, trauma, etc., your communication will change naturally without it needing to be forced.

There is a dictum that 90% of what one *experiences* one remembers, and 90% of what one *learns* one forgets. Language cannot substitute for experience, and this is one reason that quotes and vignettes are used to illustrate principles. Admittedly, anecdotes have no statistical significance and, as such, may well be (and should be) viewed with scientific distrust. Still, they create an experience, make a point, and often indicate the direction for future exploration.

Unlike medical practice where risk reduction is emphasized, creativity is needed in communication, and this always involves risk. Since this book questions widely accepted norms, challenges the status quo, attempts to reclaim healing as a mainstream medical practice, offers innovative concepts, and crosses boundaries between medicine and other professions, it role-models creative risk.

As suggested in the Frontispiece, by all means critically examine and destructure what you read here. See if it resonates. Discuss the chapters with others, and adapt the principles articulated in it to your unique circumstances. Please excuse generalizations. They are made with awareness that they do not necessarily apply to everyone and every situation.

Specific themes to listen for are expanded upon since knowing *what to listen for* is essential to professional communication. Some psychotherapy techniques are included more to raise your awareness of what is possible and to stimulate your further exploration than to suggest that you practice them untrained.

Since listening is the essence of communication, more attention is paid to it than any other aspect of communication. In fact, listening and communication are treated as being virtually synonymous.

Finally, please note that this book is intended for all healthcare practitioners. Having said that, you will see that I direct my attention primarily toward physicians. This is because I am a physician, and I am basing this book on my personal experience and research of the medical literature. Nevertheless, the principles articulated are universal, and I am personally committed to the removal of artificial barriers between professional disciplines. We are all in this work together, and have much to learn from one another.

References

1 *New York Times* (2001) Healthcare: the sound and the fury. 16 December.

2 Jenkins H (2002) The morning after. *JAMA.* **287**: 161–2.

3 *Medical Economics* (2001) What doctors want most. 17 December.

4 Beckman H, Markakis K, Suchman A *et al.* (1994) The doctor–patient relationship and malpractice. Lessons from plaintiff depositions. *Arch Intern Med.* **154**: 1365–70.

5 Sullivan P, Buske L (1998) Results from CMA's huge 1998 physician survey point to a dispirited profession. *CMAJ.* **159**: 525–8.

6 Hickson G, Federspiel C, Pichert J *et al.* (2002) Patient complaints and malpractice risk. *JAMA.* **287**: 2951–7.

7 *Newsweek* (1999) The silent anguish of the healers. 13 September.

8 Frank A (2002) *At the Will of the Body: reflections on illness.* Mariner Books, New York, NY.

9 Rowe M (2002) *The Book of Jesse: a story of youth, illness and medicine.* Francis Press, Washington DC.

10 Larson E, Yao X (2005) Clinical empathy as emotional labor in the patient–physician relationship. *JAMA.* **293**: 1100–6.

11 Ashbury F, Iverson D, Kralj B (2001) Physician communication skills: Results of a survey of general/family practitioners in Newfoundland. *MEO.* **6**: 1. www. med-ed-online.org (accessed 27 June 2005).

12 Fallowfield L, Jenkins V, Farewell V *et al.* (2002) Efficacy of a Cancer Research UK communication skills training model for oncologists: a randomized controlled trial. *Lancet.* **359**: 6506.

13   Stevens JO (1973) *Awareness: Exploring, Experimenting, Experiencing.* Bantam, New York.

14   Frankl V (1967) *The Doctor and the Soul.* Bantam, New York.

15   May GG (1987) *Will and Spirit.* HarperCollins, New York.

16   Levinson W, Cohen M, Brady D *et al.* (2001) To change or not to change: 'Sounds like you have a dilemma'. *Ann Intern Med.* **135**: 386–91.

17   Davis-Floyd R (2004) Midwifery today. www.midwiferytoday.com (accessed 27 June 2005).

1

The problem: *'it's just a lack of time'*

Having a great time. Wish I were here.
Jack Kornfield, *Postcards from the Edge*

Myth: inadequate communication is due to lack of time.

At my workshops and lectures, physicians invariably respond, 'Of course I'd listen more; it's just a lack of time.'

In this day and age, who can argue with that? Not just physicians, all healthcare professionals are scurrying as never before. Patients are admitted and discharged from hospital at a dizzying pace. Physicians hear the whip being cracked to see more patients for the same reimbursement. Those aiming for 'a more balanced life' face the painful dilemma of either cramming the same number of patients into a shorter work week (and in the process being even more pressured), or working longer hours and having less free time.

There is little empty space in the lives of most physicians and obviously there is little time for listening – a natural conclusion, except that lack of time is not the real problem. With some notable exceptions, problematic communication is more about *quality* than quantity, as the following examples demonstrate.

Absence of communication

Michael Rowe, a Yale University sociology professor, wrote a heart-rending book about his 19-year-old son Jesse's harrowing ordeal with two liver transplants and a perforated bowel that ultimately resulted in his death after months of suffering.[1] During this entire period, Michael took a leave of absence from work to be at the bedside and care for his son. Following Jesse's death, Michael was shocked when the surgeon, whom he had spoken to almost ever day over this entire period, never called to offer his condolences. What he experienced was absolute silence – and bills addressed to his deceased son.

Inappropriate communication

Attempting to educate

Annie developed type 1 diabetes. Her physician wanted to impress upon her the dangers of this disease, so he showed her pictures of gangrene and amputated limbs. He also warned her that she would be dead by the age of 35. Annie was 10 years old at the time.

Signaling gross insensitivity

David suffered from acne rosacea, which caused his nose to swell like a ripe strawberry. Being extremely sensitive about his appearance even with physicians, he finally plucked up courage and went to see a plastic surgeon. After anxiously waiting half an hour, the doctor arrived and was hardly in the room when he blurted, 'What a honker!' David's wife had to restrain him from fleeing from the humiliation.

Signaling lack of empathy

Marla required an emergency caesarian section at 25 weeks of gestation. The baby suffered major brain damage, and for three days Marla went through 'hell' as she pleaded for the medical team to discontinue life support. Short of sleep, exhausted and grieving, all her energy was focused on relieving the pain and suffering of her baby as he bled into his brain.

Her obstetrician's only comment during this time was 'Don't worry; your next one will be fine.'

The baby finally died. Deep in mourning, Marla returned for a routine post-operative visit. The obstetrician walked into the examination room and, without a single expression of regret at the baby's death, ripped off the dressings. Addressing Marla's abdomen, she remarked, 'Your scar is healing nicely.' Now, almost five years later Marla still bears deep emotional scars, and remains furious at the bizarre callousness of her physician.

Signaling hostility

Robin, an engineer, required emergency triple-bypass surgery. Post-operatively, he wanted to know the technical details of his surgery. The physician assistant's response was to snap, 'You ask a lot of questions, don't you?'

Signaling pessimism

Janice considered herself a failure when her first delivery ended in a caesarian section. She now very much wanted this second delivery to be natural. The obstetrician's opinion was that she could not deliver naturally, but he reluctantly agreed to an extension of another hour or two. Her midwife, hearing how important it was for her to succeed on her own, took the opposite position. She used empowering language saying, 'You *can* deliver naturally. Stop that negative tape that says *I can't*, and replace it with one that says *I can*.' Janice delivered successfully, and was effusively grateful. 'This was such a healing experience, I no longer feel inadequate,' she cried.

Misplacing emotion

Ever since he could remember, Eric could never run as far or as fast as other children. Now, as a 50-year-old, his exercise tolerance was even more impaired. Over the years, he went to see several physicians, and finally one ordered an echocardiogram. The findings suggested a condition known as asymmetric septal hypertrophy. The doctor did not seem unduly concerned, but referred him to a cardiologist.

One look at the echocardiogram, and the cardiologist screamed at Eric, 'What have you been doing, man! Don't you know you can drop dead at any moment from this!'

Later, the cardiologist explained that his anger had been meant for the physicians who had failed to make the correct diagnosis. Too late; his words were now indelibly imprinted on Eric's brain.

Signaling arrogance

When Philip brought some health information downloaded from the internet to his routine appointment, his internist glared at him. 'Who is the doctor in this case, you or me?' he asked.

Signaling familiarity

Andrea, an obstetrician, was examining a patient who had sustained a third-degree vaginal tear during a difficult delivery. She was pleased that the wound had finally healed. When asked what it looked like down there, Andrea, thinking that she had a very good rapport with the patient, replied, 'It's healed really well, but I would not recommend posing for *Playboy*.'

The patient sued.

Offering attempted humor

Charles was a jovial, resilient elderly man who always saw the positive. When his beloved wife of 40 years marriage died, he soon remarried, but his second wife died just 3 years later. His third wife did not live very much longer. All his marriages had been happy. His physician, on the other hand, felt miserable and trapped in his. When told of the death of Charles's third wife, the physician quipped, 'Do you think you can lend me your bed?' Charles was not amused.

These examples have several things in common.

- They illustrate communications that wound rather than heal.
- They are recalled years later by patients who remain angry and upset.
- The errors are not subtle.
- They demonstrate insensitivity and lack of empathy.
- Their impact is underestimated by the practitioner.

and ...

- They are primarily not caused by lack of time.

These examples are anecdotal, and yet there is plenty of evidence that many physicians listen poorly, miss vital non-verbal clues, misdiagnose emotional and mental conditions, and respond with a lack of understanding and insight.

Physicians often express the sentiment that all we need to do to satisfy patients is to listen longer. There is no evidence for this at all. In fact, the experience of time is highly subjective, so that a few minutes of attentive listening feels much longer to the speaker than multitasked distracted listening.

What is needed is *better* communication more than *longer* communication. Yes, there are times when patients do need more time; yes, and physicians should be reimbursed for these situations. On the other hand, the satisfaction that results from time freely given to patients can be immeasurable.

Practice points

Notice how the words in the anecdotes above wound rather than heal. Except for the occasional lonely soul, most people prefer not to be dealing with health issues and the healthcare system. If for no other reason than this, it is a safe assumption that *all* patients are emotionally traumatized by their illness or disability. In your encounter with patients, you have the power to either add to the trauma or help heal it. How you listen and respond largely determines the difference. There is no third alternative. It's as simple as that.

- Listening can never hurt, but words can. If in doubt of what to say, be silent. Remember, unless your words hurt, you will be remembered much longer for your listening than your speaking.
- Silence is in fact a very powerful communication tool even if it begins to feel uncomfortable to you as you wait for the patient to speak. Idle chatter and premature words of comfort and reassurance stifle insight and meaningful dialogue. Therapists frequently use silence to stimulate their clients to reach deeply inside.
- Always pause momentarily before responding to a patient. You may have something funny, or angry, or caustic, or judgmental, or potentially shaming to say, and this moment of pausing will give you time to reflect on the way your comment is likely to be received.
- Notice the tone of your voice. Tone is as important as the words you use. Much that is communicated goes through the right (emotional) brain rather than the left (linear, intellectual, verbal) brain. Practice modulating your tone of voice. This seemingly simple step can make a big difference.
- Should a patient express strong emotion or concern, avoid denial or defensiveness. Ask questions in a calm voice until you are sure you fully understand not only the relevant facts but also the underlying emotions. Respond back, verifying that you have indeed grasped the essence of the communication.
- Empathy can never hurt. Consciously find an opportunity to respond empathetically at least once in any encounter.

Reference

1   Rowe M (2002) *The Book of Jesse: a story of youth, illness and medicine*. Francis Press, Washington DC.

2

Seeing the whole

At medical school I learned to repair violins.
It took many more years for me to hear their music.

The author

'How many sore throats do you think I treated in my career?' the retired pediatrician asked rhetorically. 'None,' he continued, 'I treated patients, not sore throats.'

Sir William Osler (1849–1919) said essentially the same thing, 'The good physician treats the disease; the great physician treats the patient who has the disease.'

Skilled treatment of disease is the basis of good medical care and this is a precondition to any attempts at healing. Exceptional medical care demands that pathology not be approached as freestanding and unrelated to the person who has the pathology. One woman facing the prospect of a hysterectomy protested her impersonal care to her gynecologist. 'I am not just a uterus on legs!' she exclaimed.

The division between the roles of patient and healthcare professional is to some extent artificial. We are all patients, if not now, certainly sooner or later. Patients are human too. They/we have hopes, fears, losses, suffering. They/we also have aspects of self that are healthy and resilient. Excellent care requires that the disease be treated, contained, and possibly eradicated, AND that the person with the disease be assisted to heal, i.e., be restored to health or *wholeness*.

Currently, patients come to the medical establishment for treatment and to the alternative community for healing. This creates a split or division of care that is inherently unhealthy, and denies both patients and practitioners the symbiotic benefits that are possible. Healing combined with treating creates an effect that is greater than the sum of their parts.

Maimonides, the 12th-century physician, understood this concept of integrated care very well. He wrote: 'The physician should make every effort to see that everyone, sick and healthy alike, should always be cheerful, and he should seek to relieve them of the spiritual and psychological forces that cause anxiety. This is the first principle in curing any patient.'[1]

With the development of scientific medicine and the explosion of technology, contemporary medicine has distanced from the care of the patient in favor of the treatment of disease. Similarly, mainstream medicine has largely abandoned the word *heal*, except to use it to describe the repair of a specific body part, e.g., 'the fracture has healed' or 'the laceration has healed'. The lay public and the alternative therapy community have, on the other hand, embraced the term and now use it sometimes indiscriminately to describe treatment, e.g., 'the breast cancer is healed'; *or* any modality that offers comfort and support, e.g., 'healing yoga candle lighting in the park'.

In order to reclaim the word *heal* with any degree of specificity, as in *Communication Skills that Heal*, it is useful to dwell on semantics – clarifying terminology and concepts that are frequently confusing.

The terms *hole, whole, heal, healing, healer,* and *holy* are related. The original Old English word for *heal* is *haelen* from the Old High German *heilen* – to heal. The word *holy* is similarly derived from the Old English *halig* meaning whole.[2] There is an inverse relationship between healing and trauma – they are flip sides of the coin as will become apparent later.

Clarification of terms

Whole

Imagine a perfectly healthy, unflawed human being totally unified in mind, body, and spirit – a rosy-cheeked infant unblemished in any way, or an Adonis-like Greek sculpture of the ideal human figure. This individual is *whole* – a unified, intact, complete, fully functioning *universe* of atoms numbering approximately 10×27th power. In health, the estimated 10–100 trillion cells that comprise the human body function as a seamless whole. Emerging from this universe of cells and suffusing it are thoughts, feelings, spirit, and consciousness. Mindbodyspirit are indivisible.

Hole

Trauma in one form or another sooner or later strikes and creates a *hole* or split within the *whole*. A piece of the whole is lost. Trauma is always associated with losses, and disease, which is a form of trauma, is therefore associated with losses that are not only physical, but also psychological and spiritual. Some examples of losses include loss of function, income, security, well-being, sense of invulnerability, power, and control.

Healing

To heal is to mend. The individual yearns to become whole again. Healing is therefore aimed at the restoration of wholeness or healthy function. The organism that has been traumatized has to reorganize around the existing hole, incorporate losses, release tension, and restore continuity and function. Since health is unlikely to be perfect, healing does not restore perfection, rather it aims at maximum restoration of healthy function in the current situation. If the trauma has been severe, often an internal scar remains, to be revealed in times of stress.

Healing of an organism is never absolute so that there is no such state as *being completely healed*. Even as one trauma is being healed, another is being inflicted. Like the layers of an onion or an archeological site, once one aspect of self is healed, another layer of woundedness is exposed that can be healed.

Healing is difficult to define. My working definition relative to medicine is:

Healing is the ever-deepening process of bringing together or integrating that which is split or separated in an individual so that all aspects of that individual function as one, in harmony with self and environment.

Healer

In a certain sense, the term *healer* is a misnomer. All organisms are designed to heal spontaneously, i.e., are self-healing. The role of the healer is to remove impediments that retard healing.

Sir William Osler might have reflected this more specifically had he said, 'The good physician treats the disease; the great physician treats the disease *and helps heal* the patient who has the disease.'

This concept of healer can be better understood through the use of metaphor.

Imagine a trauma that results in a fairly large skin wound. Exudate seeps from the wound and forms a thick hard scab that protects the delicate tissue from exposure to the elements. New skin grows in from the edges and base of the wound. This new tissue encounters the scab (or foreign body, or infection) and cannot grow further. The healer's job here is to debride the wound; to remove the scab that interferes with healing.

In the realm of spirit or emotion, expressions of grief form the first stage of healing. The expression: 'tears are nature's way of washing the wound' refers to this. Sometimes grief and mourning is interrupted and healing is premature or incomplete.

Continuing the metaphor, incomplete healing results in 'scar tissue', and emotional scarring may require 'supportive debridement' in the form of therapy or listening.

Health

Understanding and defining health is remarkably difficult.

The WHO in 1948 defined health as 'A state of complete, physical, mental and social well-being and not merely the absence of disease or infirmity.'[3] This definition has remained unchanged.

'Complete' well-being – huh? Think back on the times that you have been suffused by a feeling of complete well-being – when you felt complete, contented, and totally not wanting anything to be different. If your experience is similar to mine, these moments are uncommon, delicious, and fleeting. The implication of the WHO definition is that health is extraordinary.

Well-being in turn is defined as: 'The state of being happy, *healthy*, or prosperous.'[4]

This is a circular definition since we have seen that health is considered dependent on well-being, and well-being is dependent on being healthy.

Rather than attempting to define health, it is easier to list the characteristics of health. Health and well-being are probably best thought of as relative rather than absolute phenomena – aspirations rather than accomplishments.

Holistic

The object of holistic medicine is to treat the whole system rather than individual components of it with the awareness that the gestalt of the whole is greater than a simple totaling of the individual parts, i.e., the 'system' itself adds something additional. Another way of stating this, the *unity* of *mindbodyspirit* is not simply *mind + body + spirit* and a holistic prescription is more than:

- *for spiritual health do x*
- *for emotional health do y*
- *for physical health do z*
- $x + y + z =$ complete health.

This approach oversimplifies and divides what is an integrated whole. Humans are studied scientifically through division. This is the nature of science after all. Excellent practice, however, requires that there be a clear awareness that this division of the body into systems is artificial and done mainly for convenience.

Unfortunately, the term *holistic* has also become tainted by those practitioners who direct their energy towards the promotion of 'natural' products, herbs, quartz crystals, healing ointments, and other therapies of questionable merit – most of which have nothing to do with restoration of wholeness. A practitioner who hands out a packet of herbs, for example, is no more holistic than one handing out a packet of pills.

Holy work

The same work that is considered 'holy' can also be exploitative and mundane. The difference lies in the motivation behind the activity. If the primary aim of medical practice is to create healing, and the work is conducted ethically with the patient's well-being in mind, then it is holy. I also think of work that is done above and beyond that which is expected or reimbursed as holy – acts of kindness, consideration, special effort, etc. The term *holy* need not have a religious connotation.

The relationship of healing to trauma

This can be summed up by the following adaptation of a commonly used expression, i.e., 'Life is a beach and then you die.'

I love walking on the beach. Sometimes there is less sand than at other times. The nature of a beach is to be subject to constant wave action that erodes it then replenishes it. Sand and water are in dynamic interaction. Sometimes a major storm or hurricane strikes and upsets this delicate balance overwhelming the beach and perhaps irrevocably damaging it. In other situations, there may be a steady erosion of beach without the return of sand, and the beach disappears.

Life is like a beach subject to tidal action in that it consists of an endless cycle of traumas and healings; sand and water in dynamic relationship, and optimally in balance. This process is not sequential, so that at any one time healing of one aspect of self may take place while trauma to another occurs.

For some, a constant erosion of spirit and emotion occurs without replenishment, e.g., a self-neglecting healthcare professional; the caregiver of an Alzheimer patient; a patient with a chronic relapsing illness, etc.; and the result is depletion or burnout. Others describe this erosion differently. Just as the bloodstream requires nutrients, the *soulstream* requires its own form of nourishment. Effective care requires attention to both (Rabbi Goldie Milgram, personal communication).

As in the case of a beach that is struck by an occasional major storm or tsunami, a person may be hit by a life-threatening traumatic event that results in death, injury, or post-traumatic stress disorder (PTSD).

Peter Levine, the trauma expert, described serious trauma in a workshop as 'an internal straightjacket created when a devastating moment is frozen in time.' This description vividly describes serious trauma as not only creating a hole, but also embodying or creating a fixity or rigidity that permanently interferes with smooth functioning of the individual and inhibits adaptation to changing circumstances.

Healing modalities

Major trauma impacts on the health and well-being of the entire individual – mind, body and soul. Injury is never limited to a single dimension of self. Since the *whole* is affected, it follows then that treatment inevitably needs to be holistic.

This contrasts with prevailing medical practice. Medical treatment is usually accompanied by problem-solving explanation, counsel and advice. This is important but, on its own, not enough. To be holistic, the practitioner must take into account the very real emotional and reptilian components of the patient's mind – not just the intellectual left-brained component responsible for conscious thought and speech. We are much more than simply the thoughts we hold. The late Israeli poet Zelda expressed it well: 'My soul says: Facts are a wall around the self.'

The expression: *understanding everything, changing nothing* sums up the effect of a purely intellectual approach. Attempts to find meaning or make sense of trauma may in fact inhibit healing and is one explanation being offered for why humans are prone to PTSD and not animals. For healing to occur, analysis and intellectual processing may have to be interrupted so that deeply rooted emotions can be expressed.

All healing work tends to follow a certain predictable path:

- It circumvents the left brain *thinking about* state, and supports the spirit, evokes emotion, raises awareness, and integrates experience.
- It brings the individual into the *present* – important, since healing does not take place in the past or the future, but in the here and now.
- It connects with the senses. Guided imagery, music, dance, drumming, art, poetry, writing, touch, body work, smell – all modalities are used to connect with the senses, stimulate awareness, and influence the right brain.

- Healing does not occur in isolation, it emerges from a healing relationship. Communication heals when it provides safety, support, relief of isolation, encourages the retelling of the trauma story, reflects back the best self of the individual, reminds the patient of his/her identity besides that of patient, and supports the processing and integration of emotion. In other words – it includes speaking and is more than simple articulation – it requires relationship.

The act of being listened to in a deep way is inherently profoundly healing. It feels almost visceral, and Dan Bloom refers to this when he says, 'I touch by my listening' (personal communication).

Practice points

Distinguish between study and practice

- A successful *student* divides and organizes material into manageable portions for purposes of study and understanding.
- A successful *practitioner* appreciates that the healthy body functions as a seamless whole.

Practice seeing the whole

As a healthcare professional, your radar screen is naturally set to spot and treat disease. Basically, what makes you a good physician tends to make you a poor healer; practice backing off to see the bigger picture, i.e., what do I know about the life, stresses, and supports of the patient who has the disease?

- Use the problem list in the medical chart to note your patients' primary relationships and personal interests. Even the most seemingly uninspired patient has some unique interest, as I found out one day when a patient with prostate cancer revealed his hobby was collecting martini swizzle sticks!
- Use Post-it notes in the chart to record events of personal significance in the life of your patient, e.g., 'Taking first cruise next month.' This way you will remember to inquire about the vacation at a later visit.
- Remind your patients, particularly those with chronic illnesses, 'You are much more than your disease.' This way, they are reminded of their identities beyond the disease process. This is accomplished through your recognition of who they are, and your personal interactions with them.

Ask 'How are you?', rather than 'How is your knee (or back or cough, etc.)?' In doing this you address the person rather than the disease.

Acknowledge those present in the room, since they are an extension of your patient and possibly a valuable support.

One mother brought her very active child in for a well-infant visit. The pediatrician noted, 'Your child is fine, but how are you? You look tired?' She explained how difficult it was to put her son to bed at night. In a few minutes he gave her a strategy and within 2 days her son had been trained.

Allow your patients to see that you are more than a physician

Expand your own areas of interest. The more literature you read, art you view, sport you watch, adventures or travel you experience, the more interesting you will be to your patients and the more interesting they will seem to you. Your patients benefit from your personal development.

The way you decorate your office says something about *you*. Patients look at the photos of your family on your desk; drawings of your children framed on your walls. Do not be afraid to reveal your personality, but do this consciously and professionally. When you take a vacation resist the practice of some physicians to have their receptionists say they are at a conference. Your patients are smarter than that; they'll spot your suntan. Besides, it's fine to take a vacation. It indicates you are human and models self-care.

Find a comfortable balance between deconstructing your image as an authority figure (so patients don't expect perfection) while retaining your patients' confidence that you are trustworthy and in control.

Practice viewing the world with binocular vision

With 'one eye' look for *pathology*, and with the other look for *health*. In other words, not only see what is wrong with a situation or your patient, but also look for what is right – and support it. Follow former President Clinton's example when in his 1993 inaugural address he said, 'There is nothing wrong with America that cannot be cured by what is right with America.'

An 87-year-old man saw a cardiologist for symptoms of cardiac failure. 'What do you expect,' the physician commented. 'You had bypass surgery 12 years ago, and your heart valve is leaking. There is nothing we can do for you.' Four years later, now aged 91, he was still vibrant and an important member of the family. His physician had failed to note that this patient had a toughness and resiliency greater than most, and as a result had neglected to support this patient's strengths.

Apply the *Healing Plan*

When using the SOAP formula (Subjective, Objective, Assessment, Plan), consider having two Plans – one that is formulated for *treatment* (of the disease) and the other for *healing* (of the patient). Most patients require both. For example, a patient with arthritis of a knee might need treatment with an anti-inflammatory medication, physical therapy, and a cane. A healing plan would have the practitioner inquire about losses – self-esteem, function, mobility, activities, and asking what would be needed to restore maximum function considering the limitations imposed by the arthritis.

In some situations, there is little or no place for healing, e.g., a medical emergency. In other situations, e.g., terminal illness, active treatment may have little to offer.

Avoid the usual pitfalls of healing

Confusing healing with treating

- Treatment is goal-oriented towards cure. Healing is process-oriented towards wholeness.
- Treatment is directed towards solving someone's problem. Healing is directed towards being on the journey with someone.
- Treatment focuses on pathology. Healing focuses on both pathology and health.
- Treatment introduces solutions. Healing removes impediments.
- Treatment is sometimes possible. Healing is always possible.
- Treatment is applied by another. Healing emerges from relationship.
- With treatment, the patient is generally passive. With healing, the patient is an active participant.

- With treatment the recipient experiences powerlessness. With healing, the recipient experiences empowerment.
- Treatment is unidirectional – it benefits the patient. Healing benefits both, and enhances the well-being of both healer and patient.

Confusing healing with comforting

Healing involves mourning and integrating loss. It is often a painful experience. Anyone who has been through serious psychotherapy can relate to this. As a result, many avoid the work of healing, and choose instead to be comforted and to move on hoping that time will heal.

Sweet ritual, holding of hands, lighting of candles etc. may be comforting and relieve isolation but, unless it facilitates deep mourning process and the integration of loss, it may actually impede healing.

Seeking premature healing

Following a trauma it is human nature to want an end to suffering. Frequently there is a rush to healing in the hope of 'creating closure' or 'putting the event behind us.' As a result, much needed integration and reorganization of self around the trauma is overlooked. Healing cannot be forced.

References

1   Rambam (Rabbi Moshe Ben Maimon, Maimonides, 1135–1204) from *Hanhagat HaBriut*, The regimen of healthcare. www.azamra.org/Heal/Resources/Rambam.html (accessed 27 June 2005).

2   www.etymonline.com/index.php?term = holy (accessed 27 June 2005).

3   www.who.int/about/definition/en/ (accessed 27 June 2005).

4   Falk M (2002) About facts. In: *The Spectacular Difference: Selected Poems Zelda*. Hebrew Union College Press, Cincinnati, OH. http://ag.arizona.edu/futures/home/glossary.html (accessed 27 June 2005).

3

Resistance

The dogmas of the quiet past are inadequate to the stormy present.
Abraham Lincoln

Oh how I lectured, cajoled, entreated, encouraged, supported, cheerled, and yes, even bribed Bessie to lose weight. I offered to credit her office bill with $10 for every pound she lost. My arguments were rational and flawless, 'You will feel more comfortable, your leg ulcers will heal, your diabetes, high blood pressure and breathing will all improve.' She listened respectfully, smiled sweetly, agreed with me, yet her weight continued to hover in the high 300 lb range.

Eventually Mindy, Bessie's daughter, joined forces with me. She emptied the house of all food and delivered a daily 1200 calorie food ration. Bessie soon slimmed down enough to be able to drive to the supermarket and then . . . .

Bessie died weighing close to 400 lb. Her family asked me to be a pallbearer at the funeral. They knew I had tried my best. Despite all logic and good intentions, something had kept her on a course of self-destruction.

In every medical practice there are emphysematous patients who keep smoking, diabetics who indulge in rich desserts, workaholics who keep working, couch potatoes who watch television all day – and physicians who don't listen. Something keeps them, and us, from changing. At least smokers can attribute their behavior to addiction. As for obese patients, genetic and metabolic factors play a role. The question remains, *why is it so difficult to change behavior that is obviously harmful to ourselves and perhaps others?*

General Norman Swartzkopf is attributed to have said, 'The truth of the matter is that you *always* know the right thing to do. The hard part is doing it.' In other words, intellectual knowledge does not necessarily translate to change in behavior.

Obituaries of experts in the field of human behavior hint at their struggles.

- Wayne Oats who coined the term *workaholic* wrote 57 books by the time he died.
- Herbert Freudenberger, who identified and labeled the condition of *burnout*, worked 15 hours a day until 3 weeks before his death.
- Meyer Friedman who wrote the book *Type A Personality and Your Heart* had type A personality.

Resistances

There are many factors that combine to create resistance to change – even change for the better. In this chapter I want to focus just on one, since I believe that this particular factor plays a major role in limiting effective communication in the medical profession.

This factor is *resistance* or more commonly referred to as defense mechanism. This is not to be confused with the regular use of the word resistance, so it is italicized here.

Resistance is a Gestalt therapy term that refers to the intrapersonal interference that prevents an individual from completing an action that satisfies a need.

The following is a simple example.

John's wife complains that when they have a disagreement he shuts down and she finds this very exasperating. His silence threatens their relationship. Working in therapy, he finds a connection with his clamming up as an adult and a pattern of behavior that he developed as a child. In his single-parent family, only his mother was allowed to speak up; children were to be seen and not heard. John learned this important lesson unconsciously at a very young age and this enabled him to fit in with his family. As an adult, this survival mechanism persisted and became a handicap. Only during therapy did he discover how many of his female adult relationships had been ruined by this attitude.

Introjection

The above is an example of one form of *resistance*, termed introjection. In this case the introject is *that silence is preferable to speaking up.*

With introjection, information is unconsciously incorporated into one's psyche. This information is unexamined and unprocessed in the manner of a baby swallowing milk without chewing and tasting it to see if it is appetizing. Hence, a child internalizes values of parents, teachers, and society, and emulates them. This information is valuable since it allows for survival and integration with community. Inevitably misinformation creeps in as well, and may set up the individual for a lifetime of dysfunctional behavior, prejudice, and perhaps low self-esteem. A little boy who is called 'disorganized and messy' by his mother may retain this as an introject forever, resisting all attempts by others to enforce some structure on him. His response is always 'I am not an organized person.'

> The introjector minimizes differences between what he is swallowing whole and what he might truly want if he was allowed to make this discrimination. He thereby neutralizes his own existence by avoiding the aggressiveness required for destructuring what exists. It is as if anything which exists is inviolate; he is not to change it; he must take it all as it comes.[1]

Introjects are our 'truths'. They are so deep-seated that it takes profound moments of insight to reveal them and to integrate new ways of thinking. One of the problems of introject and other forms of *resistance* occurs when we or our environment change, and these *resistances* have outlived their survival usefulness. The *resistances* then sabotage healthy new behavior. We cannot force our *resistances* to disappear; however, when they are brought to our conscious awareness and we develop other more useful ways of functioning, then we lessen our dependency on them.

The chief medical resident eats on the run; takes notes while he listens to his patients; speaks on his cell phone while he drives. He is an incessant multitasker. One day, I am asked to present a lunchtime workshop on stress, and choose to let the audience finish their meal before I begin. As he begins to reprimand me for not beginning on time, he suddenly becomes wide-eyed as he recalls that his father — an internist — was always late for meals, eating on the run and never present to the family.

In this example, the chief resident had introjected that multitasking was normal behavior for a physician. Until this deeply rooted myth had been unearthed, he was unwilling to alter his behavior.

The biblical book of Exodus in the bible has a story related to introject when it tells of a former slave who collected sticks on the Sabbath despite an edict that this act was punishable by death. One interpretation of the story is that as a former slave this man had introjected that it was normal to work every day and could not change his behavior.

Medical students introject as they absorb vast amounts of material in their training, and integrate as norms of their profession the behavior of their mentors and authority figures. Being good students, they are particularly vulnerable to introjecting incorrect information as well. Lessons become 'truths' as they are handed down from generation to generation of physicians.

Many of these core beliefs interfere with self-care, relationship, and communication. In subsequent chapters we will examine them and see which need to be spat out and replaced. There are other forms of *resistance* besides introject.

Projection

With *projection*, the issue or quality or locus of control is projected away from the self onto something else, e.g., saying, 'The room is very hot' instead of 'I am feeling very hot.' Similarly, 'The donut is very tempting' instead of 'I am craving a donut and I know I have had two already.' A problem in relationship occurs when we project our feelings onto others, e.g., 'Oh dear, you must feel so sad ...' when the other does not feel sad but rather feels angry. The sadness is a projection of the listener. Patients may unconsciously project qualities onto the physician that prevent the physician being seen for who he is, e.g., father, authority figure, teacher, rescuer, etc. Similarly, as practitioners we may project qualities onto our patients. Based on personal experience we may, for example, either see an elderly patient as senile or as filled with wisdom of age when neither is reality.

Confluence

With *confluence*, individuals prematurely agree as a way of avoiding conflict. The excessively smiling, agreeable, yet recalcitrant patient is probably being confluent — as is the ideal 'good patient'. The problem with a confluent patient like Bessie is that one is not likely to connect with him or her on a deeper level. Consequently, one cannot know what she is truly thinking or feeling.

Deflection

With *deflection*, individuals avoid confrontation by deflecting issues, e.g., humor can be used to deflect pain and suffering, as in the case of the stereotypical comic or clown. Patients too may deflect underlying emotions with angry outbursts or excessive humor or smiling.

Practice points

- At first sight, the patient who speaks continuously seems to be open and revealing. Actually, the opposite is true. Insight rarely emerges from excessive talking which protectively keeps painful emotions at bay. Basically, this talk avoids true communication and it is only when chatter settles down and contact is made with underlying emotion that true communication begins. Try sitting in comfortable silence with someone, and notice what emerges.
- *Resistances* operate on an unconscious level and it is difficult to notice one's own. Take note if you frequently crack jokes or make puns (deflection); act excessively agreeably or avoid confrontation at all costs (confluence); form quick opinions of what others are thinking without asking them (projection).
- Listening frequently reveals *resistance* in others. The 'should' word is an absolute pointer to introjection, i.e., a lesson swallowed whole from an external source. When your patient for example says, 'Doctor, I know I shouldn't feel this way', interrupt by asking, 'Why shouldn't you?' This question can open up the dialogue into a discussion of what the patient really wants versus has introjected.

  'Words that don't fit the usual vocabulary of the person suggest unassimilated introjecting. Words that have flattened tone suggest that they are stand-ins for some unnamed authority' (Dan Bloom, personal communication, December 2004).
- An example of a physician's introject might be 'I'm very tired but I *shouldn't* complain – there are others less fortunate than I.' A challenge to this statement might reveal the parent or teacher that taught him to be tough at all costs, or never to complain.
- Avoid introducing introjects, e.g. *shoulding* on patients, as in telling them what they *need to* or *should* do to enhance their health. Rather reveal your concerns and invite their participation in a plan of action.
- When you ask questions as you examine, write notes while listening, record on your laptop as you hear the story – ask yourself, 'Where did I introject this multitasking behavior? Like the workaholic slave in Exodus, what learned behavior in me needs to die?'
- When you encounter resistance in another or in yourself, try not to force or pressure for change. Back off and create safety, since change is more likely to occur in an environment of safety. Embrace the valuable role that a *resistance* has played, thereby creating an environment in which it need not be utilized.

Reference

1   Polster I, Polster M (1973) *Gestalt Therapy Integrated*. Random House, New York.

4

But listening is art

Art is about freedom and control – you need both.
Sometimes doing art is like making love,
yet it's also like doing surgery.

September Heart, artist

Introject: the practice of medicine is a combination of evidence-based science and relationship-oriented art.

Everyone knows there is the art and science of medicine, right?

Higher education is always split between the liberal arts and the sciences, so this is a natural and normal division.

There is one problem. This division does not apply to the human being.

The art and science of medicine is a seemingly innocuous expression that lies at the heart of why patients feel they are not listened to or understood. This foundational belief – that medicine consists of art and science – has to be rejected if communication and healing are ever to become an integral part of medical practice.

Admittedly the phrase *art and science* has been in use for over a century, but it had a very different meaning back then. Initially, the division lay between basic disciplines such as anatomy, pathology, and bacteriology (labeled science), and the practice of medicine, e.g., therapeutics and surgery (labeled art).[1] Hence Osler's quote, 'The practice of medicine is an art, based on science.'[2]

Now this division has shifted, so basic disciplines and evidence-based medical practice fall under the rubric of science, and anything pertaining to relationship issues, i.e., spirit, emotion, communication, and healing, is relegated to the basket labeled art.

As long ago as 1888, William Draper noted the limitation of this division, astutely observing, 'We may differentiate the science from the art of medicine, but we cannot practically disassociate them.'[3]

The term *art and science of medicine* presents a significant problem for a number of reasons.

The problem of art and science

- Firstly, it is an introject – a slogan that is swallowed whole without critical examination and accepted as a truth. Once this division is held up to closer scrutiny, it becomes meaningless.
- The phrase takes something that is whole, the medical encounter, and divides it into two. It creates a boundary between two realms of practice that are in reality inseparable. If there is a perceived lack of time (as there almost always is), then art, being less imperative, tends to be glossed over.
- It encourages split thinking:
  - *I take care of treatment, someone else can handle healing.*
  - *My job is to cure you. Concerned about fees? See my business manager.*
  - *Take this medication. You are distressed by this illness? See mental health.*
- It encourages the creation of generalizations and fixed images, for example:
  - auscultation (listening to an organ) = science and utilizes technology.
  - listening (listening to the person) = art and utilizes one's natural ability. Everything labeled 'science' is considered proven and therefore must be correct, and everything labeled 'art' is anecdotal, subjective, soft, and suspect.

  A consequence of this bifurcation is that thinking becomes rigid. Banished are intuition, creativity, risk taking, curiosity, meaning, and mystery to the outermost reaches of the 'art of medicine'. Borrowing a metaphor, one frustrated patient in an orthopedic hospital exclaimed, 'Their thinking is ossified here!'
- It encourages prejudicial treatment.

  Medicine-as-science has created an explosion of knowledge and advances. This aspect of medicine is respected, financially supported, and reimbursed. Science is rigorously taught with innumerable scientific journals committed to every aspect of evidence-based medicine.

  Medicine-as-art is a stepchild, a luxury. Training is limited to an hour or two a week, and few articles on topics considered 'art' are published in medical journals. Rarely is anything considered art reimbursable in medical practice.

'This library regularly subscribes to over 2800 journals,' stated the brochure at this Ivy League medical school. This display of scientific power was impressive, even intimidating to a simple family physician. Then I had an Aha! 'How many of these journals primarily concentrate on relationship and communication?' I asked the librarian. There were none. Later I was to talk to the very harassed-sounding physician who was responsible for teaching communication skills. 'It is a minimal part of my job,' he said, 'mostly, I work in critical care.'

Notwithstanding the enlightened policy of the school the message came across loud and clear: *We are in the business of teaching science.*

With so much science needing to be ingested, it would be unrealistic to expect medical students to expand their studies of the 'art' of medicine. On the other hand, the many years of study that span the undergraduate through postgraduate training period, as long as 14 years for some, presents an ample opportunity for the teaching of relationship skills to those who plan to practice medicine versus concentrate on pure research.

- It results in sloppy science, since work that is labeled 'science' is easily accepted as such. Much of medicine that is called 'science' is in reality a function of habit, ritual, dogma, expediency, profit, and response to zealous advertising. The results are excessively high rates of medical error, inappropriate treatment, unnecessary surgery, and over-prescribing of medication.

- It results in terrible art. When encounters between practitioners and patients are videotaped they can be seen to be either smooth, efficient, relatively effortless, and comfortable, or interrupted, rushed, and clumsy. There is an aesthetic to a good encounter. The comparison with a performance is appropriate because the moment the healthcare professional enters the room, she is "on stage". All eyes and ears are glued to her performance. It is a role that needs to be carefully practiced so as to be authentic yet controlled and modulated.

- It encourages arrogance or at least the perception of arrogance. Truly brilliant scientists such as Einstein retain a sense of awe, mystery and wonder.

The divide between art and science was not always so. There was in fact a time in history when art was science, and medicine (science) was art. The ancient Greek sculptors integrated knowledge of anatomy with sensitivity to human emotion and spirit in their work. In the Middle Ages, artists kept science alive as they studied pigments, technique, light, perspective, and stained glass. During the Renaissance, Leonardo da Vinci, besides being one of the greatest artists of all time, also emerged as the first modern scientist.[4] In the 19th century, the inventor of photography, Talbot, was as much a scientist as an artist. The list is endless.

The boundary between art and science, always a fuzzy one, continues to be so today. The artist Lois Woolley said to me one day, 'I can't speak for abstract art, but one cannot be an excellent artist unless one is rigorously methodical and intelligent in one's approach' (personal communication, 2004). My response to her was, 'You sound like a scientist.'

Fred Harwin is a highly trained medical illustrator, artist, and oculist. When he is not illustrating surgical texts, he creates eyes – breathtakingly realistic prosthetic ones. The iris, with its patterns and color variations, is a marvel of complexity and uniqueness, and Fred's job is to capture it.

He does much more than this, however. He listens to his patients while he works.

Fred's practice is to have the patient spend three days with him modeling for the crafting of the new eye. This is not technically necessary, but he has found that most patients are so traumatized by the loss of their eyes that they are helped by having someone to talk to. Not only does he listen to their stories of trauma, he learns about their lives and interests.

The day I visited his laboratory, he was painting a scene of a fisherman landing a catch on the back of the eyeball. His patient, a teenager fly fisherman, was to be delighted and surprised by this. No longer would this prosthetic eye be alien to him.

Fred has a superior knowledge of anatomy. He is a superb craftsman and artist. He teaches. He listens and heals. He is a humanitarian. Which aspect of his work is science and which is art?

Should a study reveal that patients are dispirited when they lose their eyes, and regulations require that ophthalmic surgeons spend 15 minutes listening, does Fred's art now become an ophthalmologist's science?

Beautiful science is art, and highly skilled art is science. Science explains mystery, and art highlights mystery. Still, the two are indivisible, as is being increasingly appreciated. Now there is the field of neuroesthetics in which neuroscience studies the effect of art on the brain. In the field of narrative medicine, Rita Charon has demonstrated that medical students perform better academically when they write brief narratives – a creative act.[5] In other programs, students study art to assist them in their powers of observation. In workshops on communication, actors play the role of patients. I have met several medical students who are authors and artists and are determined to incorporate their art into medicine.

The true division belongs to those physicians who work with people, and those physicians whose professional lives are spent in the laboratory.

Practice points

- Accept the reality that as a scientist you have learned to divide and categorize. You have probably learned to do this very well. With this essential grounding in place, now practice zooming in on boundaries between two seemingly disparate disciplines, and see if the edges are sharp or fuzzy. What can you add to your practice by straddling boundaries?

- Challenge yourself to think beyond convention. How can you incorporate other modalities into your work? Research the use of music to soothe, raise the spirit or distract. Apply art and design to your brochures, website, etc. Invite written narratives from your patients.

> I gave my urologist friend a Walkman tape player so his patients could listen to music over headphones while he performed vasectomies. Though the procedure was painless, the sound of their tubes being clipped and cauterized was disconcerting to some. I thought this might help. He called me a few weeks later to excitedly report that his patients were so relaxed by the music that they generally fell asleep during the procedure. Now they were referring their friends to him.

Expand your appreciation of art as it reveals the human spirit. Visit art museums and spend time with individual paintings. Ask yourself, 'What was the artist thinking when he painted this or what can I tell about the subjects in the painting?'

Consider taking a creative writing class. Write your own narratives describing your medical encounters. Form small groups with your colleagues to share your material.

Most importantly once you liberate communication from its shackle as 'art', you will appreciate that it is a highly technical professional skill that can be studied as rigorously as any 'science'.

References

1 Foshay PM (1902) The new era in medicine – what it means to Cleveland. *JAMA*. **38**: 625–7.

2 www.vh.org/adult/provider/history/osler/5.html (accessed 27 June 2005).

3 Kirsner JB (2002) The most powerful therapeutic force. *JAMA*. **287**: 1909–10.

4 Atalay B (2004) *Math and the Mona Lisa: the art and science of Leonardo da Vinci.* Smithsonian Books, Washington, DC.

5 Charon R (2001) Narrative medicine: a model for empathy, reflection, professionalism, and trust. *JAMA*. **286**: 1897–902.

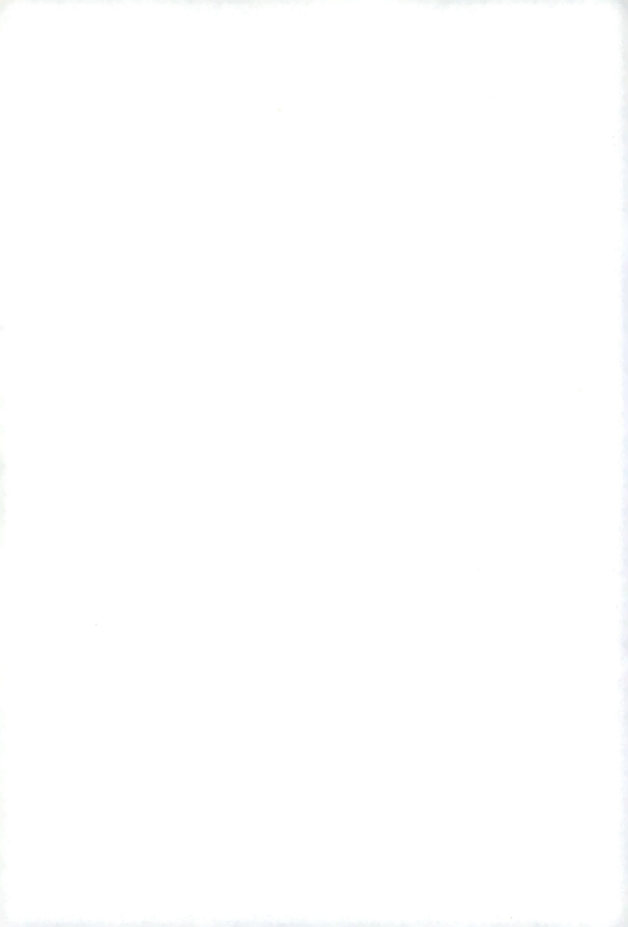

5

But there is no time for listening

If you are an administrator, listen graciously to the speech of a petitioner. Do not rebuff him before he has said all that he has planned to tell you. It is more important to a man in distress that he vent his feelings than that he win his case.

The Maxims of Ptah-hotep, 2500 BCE[1]

Introject: everyone knows that doctors are busy and do not have enough time, let alone time to listen to patients.

To study the physician's role in soliciting and developing the patient's concerns at the outset of a clinical encounter, 74 office visits were recorded. In only 17 (23%) of the visits was the patient provided the opportunity to complete his or her opening statement of concerns.[2]

Physicians solicited patient concerns in 199 interviews (75.4%). Patients' initial statements of concerns were completed in 74 interviews (28.0%). Physicians redirected the patient's opening statement after a mean of 23.1 seconds.[3]

We asked the doctors to activate a stop watch surreptitiously at the start of the communication and press it again when patients indicated that they wanted the doctor to take the lead ... Mean spontaneous talking time was 92 seconds and 78% (258) of patients had finished their initial statement in 2 minutes. Seven patients talked for longer than 5 minutes. In all cases doctors felt that the patients were giving important information and should not be interrupted.[4]

Patients know that physicians do not have enough time; why else interrupt? So do employees, hospital personnel, spouses, and children of physicians, and of course pharmaceutical representatives ('I know you are busy, doc, so if you can just quickly sign ....').

This introject about being busy is so pervasive that it seems almost inconceivable that somewhere there may exist a non-busy physician.

Most physicians do feel pressured. When asked what they want most, one-third of primary care respondents to a survey picked 'more free time'.[5] It is surprising that this figure is not even higher. One of my physician clients described her life as being: 'in perpetual rush-hour traffic with the frenetic pressure of trying to be productive in days jammed with activities and the frustration of trying to circumvent obstacles.'

Objectively, a 92-second opening statement is not a long time, but it *feels* long to someone who is rushing and has to pause to listen. The experience of time is highly subjective. Einstein referred to this with his comment, 'When a man sits with a pretty girl for an hour, it seems like a minute. But let him sit on a hot stove for a minute and it's longer than an hour. That's relativity.'[6] Always the scientist, Einstein actually tested his theory with a pretty woman, a hot stove, and a stopwatch!

In today's healthcare environment, most of the working day can be filled just carefully writing or dictating notes that satisfy the legal system, insurance, and quality control auditors.

> In a recent study of primary care physicians, it was found that they would have to spend an average of 7.4 hours a day to fully comply with preventative healthcare screening recommendations.[7]

This experience of pressure is not limited to physicians. In this speeded up information age, it applies to all segments of society including children as this advertisement for Miss Hall's School indicates:

> ... the best gifts we can give them (our children) are the gifts of time and space, time and space to become happy, curious, and accomplished, time and space to experience the joy — and not just the difficulties — of growing up.

Not only physicians, but patients too need the gift of time and space — to talk into. This is incompatible with the image of the stereotypical physician rushing from patient to patient, dictating with staccato speech, multitasking, and barely able to stop long enough to take a deep breath. There is only so much that can be crammed into a container.

Since *insufficient time* is so much part of the medical experience, one might wonder why this topic is so rarely strategically addressed.

- Why, for example, is Stephan Rechtschaffen MD, author of *Time Shifting: creating more time to enjoy your life*,[8] not a regular keynote speaker at medical meetings?

- Why do many physicians with overfilled schedules accept new patients?
- Why are so many unnecessary surgical procedures performed – ones that take up valuable time?
- Why do many heavily scheduled physicians attend lectures that are tedious and time consuming when information can be found elsewhere quicker?
- Why participate in hours of committee meetings that are of dubious value?

Yes, there are good reasons for attending lectures and sitting in on committee meetings, AND physicians have introjected that being busy, overworked, deprived of sleep, and short of time is a 'normal' part of training and practice – normal in the sense that it is virtually the norm, not normal in the sense that it is healthy or desirable. When *being busy* is accepted as normal, then there it makes no sense to seek creative solutions for being less busy.

> In a survey of 132 internal medicine house staff in a US university-based residency program, acute sleep deprivation was experienced by 34% of current house staff, and 64% were chronically sleep deprived.[9]

This is not surprising. What is somewhat startling was the finding that 'At least half of all respondents felt their sleep deprivation was *a necessary part of training*.' The authors dryly conclude, 'Education could be targeted at attitudes.' What they call attitudes, I call introjects.

Conclusion

Listening does not occur in a vacuum. It requires a solid foundation to support it. Just as a gourmet dinner is the end product of a complex and sophisticated restaurant infrastructure, listening is the end product of a well-run, well-managed practice in which time and space and structure have been created to facilitate communication. The first step involves rejecting the notion that it is normal and acceptable to live a life in which time is constantly the enemy. It also requires a commitment to the basic human right of time for adequate sleep, rest, exercise, meals, and relationship for the practitioner.

In my own practice, once I had rejected the notion that I had to be busy, I consciously worked at fine-tuning my activities, trimming away the unessential and for many years limited my work time to 32 hours per week.

Practice points

Re-evaluate your orientation towards time so that time ceases to be the enemy. If you wish to befriend time then you need to first alter your perception of it.

Experience circular time

Time is both linear – directional and goal oriented; and cyclical – the flow of holidays, seasons, anniversaries that create a rhythm and structure to a meaningful life.

Since almost all of your time will be experienced as linear it is helpful to commit to one day a week for circular time. Traditionally it has been called the Sabbath, but it need not involve religion. Develop certain rules that help to boundary it, for example no news, internet, or shopping on this day. You will probably experience this day as feeling much longer than a typical working day.

Experience more time in the present

Time involves past, present, and future. You cannot change the overall number of hours in a day. You can change how much time you spend *in the present* or *in the here and now*. The present is where all true living, healing, communicating occurs. Time in the present is expanded.

Fritz Perls described the present as 'the ever-moving zero-point of the opposites past and future'. At this point future is encountered, lived in the present, and transformed into past. In the course of a rushed day, the present becomes compressed between unfinished business of the past, and the anticipation and dwelling on the future. In practical terms, at any one moment with a patient, you may be thinking, 'I wonder if I should have handled that last patient differently,' and 'I have to remember to call Mrs X'. Not surprisingly, patients notice that you are not fully present.

Many healing practices quiet the mind and facilitate contact with the senses in the here and now. The more you are in the present, the more you begin to notice profound things. Albert Einstein said, 'He who can no longer pause to wonder and stand rapt in awe, is as good as dead; his eyes are closed.' Notice he said *stand*, not run; and that he equated being alive with being aware and in the present. Time spent thinking about past and future is time taken away from living.

Marlin Whitmer, a chaplain educator, has made the point that listening for him is reflected in the Hebrew word *hineini*, which means *here I am.* He could also alter this to *hear, I am!* To really listen requires a commitment to be present. It says to the speaker – *here, I am* (in the present) *not there* (in the future) *nor then* (in the past).

Learn to value and savor your time in the present. Develop conscious practices that support you to be here, in the room rather than: 'Having a great time, wish I were here.'

Create speed bumps in your day

Notice how life is a blur when you have spent the whole day rushing. Mini pauses of just a few seconds allow you to gather your thoughts and calm your mind and expand your day. They also facilitate your being in the present. For example, pause prior to entering the examination room. Take a deep breath and ask yourself is there any unfinished business that needs attention. If anything comes up for you, acknowledge it and park it with the understanding that you will return to the issue later. Now you can be present to your patient.

From time to time take longer breaks but rather than read or work on charts, or talk on the phone, just focus on your meal or your breathing or noticing your surroundings. You will more than make up for lost time by increased productivity from being rested.

Avoid multitasking

Multitasking is a time killer. It feels like time productively spent, but studies have shown that when attempting to do two complex tasks simultaneously, time is lost and neither task is particularly well done. In particular, it makes listening impossible, since listening is *hearing with focused attention* and your patients and others are fully aware of your inattentiveness.

Attend to FMS

Most of us have *Fear of Missing Something* syndrome. It is present when one has only one hour, and rushes through the Metropolitan Museum trying to take it all in – rather than spending that hour in one or two galleries and having a satisfying, albeit limited, experience. The irony is that the more one attempts to experience, the less one remembers.

Notice how you read your journals. Try selecting just a couple to read in depth. In *JAMA* you discover history, poetry, and art in addition to medicine. When reading a book, do it slowly, highlighting passages and making notations. Your experience will be infinitely richer. You can experience something similar lingering with people as you listen, and slowing down your interaction. The occasional patient will need more time; try to create at least one or two gaps in your schedule to allow for this.

Separate urgent from important

Most things that feel urgent are really not that important. Medical marriages are notoriously unsatisfactory because of delayed gratification – there always seems to be something more important. Prioritize your day with items that are both urgent and important as top priority.

It helps to ask yourself what you would want to read on your tombstone. Is it *He was a good physician* or *He was a good father* or *He was a good physician and father*?

One family physician did just this. He decided to co-parent his daughter when she was born, so he cut his work week down to 20 hours. Now 16 years later, she no longer needs constant parenting yet he has no intention of resuming full-time work. As for income, they have learned to live with less and are doing just fine.

Distinguish between emotional and chronological time

Though modern life has speeded up, emotional time has not changed an iota. It still takes weeks, months, even years to recover from losses. Give yourself and others the gift of space and time to integrate transitions and losses.

Utilize time as an investment

Invest time in order to save time. At first it might feel frustrating and counterproductive spending hours designing systems intended to save you time. In the long run, you will be surprised at your empowerment. You can invest time in:

- designing questionnaires, information packages, and selecting computer systems that streamline your operation and increase efficiency

- training employees to maximize their potential and improve morale
- implementing principles of total quality improvement so that quality of care improves, mistakes are reduced, and patient satisfaction is increased
- simplifying your life, reducing debt clutter, and creating space
- developing collaborative relationships so that you do not have to reinvent the wheel and coverage arrangements to maximize your time off.

Appreciate time as a non-renewable resource

Value your time and use it wisely. It is the only life you have. If your workplace does not allow you to utilize your time in a way that supports a healthy and meaningful life, then it is time to re-evaluate your career.

Re-evaluate your introject about listening and time

It is only the occasional patient who needs more than a few minutes of listening time and these patients can often be scheduled to return when it is more convenient. Remember, just by being fully in the present, you are giving your patients more time *without spending more time.*

Far from taking time, so many benefits accrue to you when you listen that in the long run, you probably experience a net gain in time. Some of the possible reasons for this are as follows:

- *Fewer malpractice lawsuits.* The decision to litigate is often associated with a perceived lack of caring and/or collaboration in delivery of healthcare.[10] Others have found that lawsuits are dependent as much on interpersonal skills as clinical ability.[11,12] Lawsuits, defensive medicine, and higher malpractice insurance premiums cost time and money.
- *Listening improves your relationships with patients, employees, colleagues, and others.* Your employees are your greatest asset and they will look after your interests and make your life easier if you show them that you care.
- *Listening is of inestimable value to your close personal relationships.* You will be amazed at how more productive you are when you are happy in your closest relationship. Besides, divorce takes time.
- *Listening improves patient care and patient satisfaction.* You will experience a free public relations bonanza when your patients rave about your abilities to listen and understand – in stark contrast to many of your colleagues. You will not have to spend time and energy promoting your

practice. As patient care improves, you will have to spend less time on unnecessary investigations and repeat patient visits.

- Satisfaction derived from the positive feedback you receive will go a long way to reducing your risk of burnout and will most likely extend your career.

Bottom line: you cannot afford *not* to listen.

References

1   Donaldson F (1959) *The Maxims of Ptah-hotep (2500 BCE)*. Vantage Press, New York.

2   Beckman HB, Frankel RM (1984) The effect of physician behavior on the collection of data. *Ann Intern Med.* **101**: 692–6.

3   Marvel MK, Epstein RM, Flowers K *et al.* (1999) Soliciting the patient's agenda. Have we improved? *JAMA.* **281**: 283–7.

4   Langewitz W, Denz M, Keller A *et al.* (2002) Spontaneous talking time at start of consultation in outpatient clinic: cohort study. *BMJ.* **325**: 682–3.

5   Rice B (2001) What doctors want most. *Med Econ.* **78**: 38–40.

6   Mirsky S (2002) Einstein's hot time. *Sci Am.* **102**: 102.

7   Yarnall KS, Pollak KI, Ostbye T *et al.* (2003) Primary care: is there enough time for prevention? *Am J Public Health.* **93**: 635–41.

8   Rechtschaffen S (1996) *Time Shifting: creating more time to enjoy your life.* Doubleday, New York.

9   Rosen IM, Bellini LM, Shea JA (2004) Sleep behaviors and attitudes among internal medicine housestaff in a US university-based residency program. *Acad Med.* **79**: 407–16.

10 Beckman HB, Markakis KM, Suchman AL (1994) The doctor – patient relationship and malpractice. Lessons from plaintiff depositions. *Arch Intern Med.* **134**: 1365–70.

11 Rice B (2003) Why some doctors get sued more than others. *Med Econ.* **80**: 73–7.

12 Hickson GB, Federspiel CF, Pichert JW *et al.* (2002) Patient complaints and malpractice risk. *JAMA.* **287**: 2951–7.

6

But listening is simple

A small hole in the body, a large hole in the soul.
Rabbi Dov Ber, the Mezritcher Magid, 1704–72

Introject: that listening does not take training and skill. Rather, it is something simple and natural.

A member of the audience raised her hand and asked, 'What does one do doctor, if a patient wants to talk about God?'

The speaker, a prominent authority on religion and medicine responded, 'Just do something simple, like listen.'

I leapt out of my seat. 'But listening is *not* simple!' I protested.

Several heads around me nodded vigorously. They knew that listening is one of the most complex, active diagnostic and therapeutic skills in the healthcare professional's repertoire.

When on a narrative medicine list serve, a chaplain claimed he was 'a simple container for the stories of patients.' I responded with the following note:

As one of those who trained with the Healthcare Chaplaincy, I was forced to confront my own apprehension at visiting the sick, armed with nothing but a book of psalms. With no stethoscope to confer authority, no white coat to hide behind, all psychotherapy techniques on hold, and my physician identity for the most part hidden, I was totally dependent on the power of *Presence* and my ability to listen. . . . My role was to bring a human connection, to establish an I–thou relationship that relieved some of this isolation which is the very essence of suffering. . . .

This required me to listen with great care and at varying times to reflect back, to inject humor, to support silence or to offer blessing or prayer. All of this was based on what I heard and my own emotional response to the narrative. Far from being a passive receptacle, this was a very, very active process.

While I displayed empathy (therapeutic validation), little was based on compassion. This, in fact, is one of the great myths of listening. Rather, I was simply doing my job, which was to listen professionally, something few physicians are trained to do. Compassion emerged from the interaction, rather than caused it.

Finally, while I heard their narrative, they heard mine – my body language, choice of words, and so forth, hence determining what they in turn chose to share.

Barry Bub MD
Advanced Physician Awareness Training

No way can professional listening ever be construed as 'simple', nor can the listener be considered a simple container. In practice most physicians listen for clues about the disease rather than the patient.

The following scenario is very typical. Here the question was whether the patient could be safely discharged.

'How's the pain Joseph?'
'Not too bad doc.'
'Bowels moving OK?'
'No problem.'
'Walking in the hall?'
'Yes.'
'We'll be sending you home tomorrow, OK?'
'OK, doc.'
'Here are your prescriptions. Be sure to schedule an appointment for follow up.'

This type of encounter occurring many thousands of times a day in hospitals can be described more as an exchange of information at the simplest level rather than as an act of professional listening. I happened to visit Joseph later in the day. It was on the first day of my chaplaincy training. Needless to say, I was feeling very insecure in this new role.

'What on earth am I doing here?' I wondered. 'I must have been crazy to sign up for this training. How do you pray with someone?' We had been given minimal direction other than to listen, and offer a prayer if the patient wanted it. The directive *You are bringing God into the room* played through my mind. 'I am?' I ruminated. 'How bizarre, I thought God was everywhere.'

Joseph, age 67, was one of my first patients. He was soon to be discharged. He had undergone back surgery 2 days previously. I reviewed his chart, noted he was diabetic, had mild hypertension, was Jewish, married, and a businessman.

Pausing momentarily at the threshold of the room, I took a deep breath and did a quick personal inventory: anxious, afraid, self-conscious, ambivalent. OK, it's the first day. Just act calm and natural, and see what evolves.

Joe was lying in bed listening to music through the headphones of his Walkman. The room was bare except for some basic furniture, a few magazines, and one small vase of flowers with a card attached. There were no visitors.

He immediately removed the headphones when he saw me enter. To me this was a welcoming gesture. His hair was thinning and gray, he was overweight, and needed a shave. He looked old for his age.

'Hello, I'm Barry Bub, chaplain today for this floor. How are you?'
'I'm doing very well, thank you. Going home tomorrow. What religion are you?' he asked, squinting at my name badge.
'I'm Jewish.'
'You are? Are you a rabbi?'
'No, I'm in chaplaincy training, I'm married to a rabbi though. Does that count?'
'Ha!' he muttered. 'You got children?'
'Yes, I have three. One ultra-orthodox, one leaning towards Christianity, and one relatively neutral.'
'As long as they are happy. And where are you from?'
'From South Africa; I have been here since 1973.'
Interesting that he is being so aggressively curious. Either he is checking me out, or perhaps he is just bored. Anyway, enough about me.
'Tell me about yourself. Why are you here?' I asked.
'I had a laminectomy. The fourth one. Two on my neck and two on my lower spine. All this from an accident in 1980.'
'You have had pain all these past 20 years?' I asked.

'Yes, I can't complain though. It's been with me all the time, but I have been fortunate. Did well in business and made enough to retire on.'

'Why can't you complain?' I asked.

'Because it was God's will. Not meant to punish me, but just God's will. I was not a good person in my time, however. Not been a good friend to anyone. I never hurt anyone though. My friends were my wife and child.'

Hmm, interesting comments.

'So no friends other than your wife and child?' I repeated back.

'No, I was withdrawn, antisocial. I had a rough childhood and then the accident. Yes, it's been a rough life. But I have my wife, child, and now grandchildren.'

'What was your childhood like?' I asked.

'Very rough. Food, clothing, school, that's it.'

'So a roof over your head, and basics, that's all,' I continued, hoping to encourage him.

'Yes' he replied.

'No love, affection, and support,' I added, emphasizing his point.

'No, but I did give to my wife and child.'

'Just to your immediate family, no one else?'

'No, I've never trusted anyone.'

Pause.

'And no one knew that there was a loving side to you?'

'No,' he replied, wiping away a tear. 'I just want to recover from surgery, live 10 more years then I'll be ready to meet my Maker. Now tell me about yourself . . . '

This must be very significant; he is changing the subject.

'No, I'm really interested in hearing more about you. One day I'll be a patient and I hope someone will be there to listen to me.'

   Just then a male nurse walked into the room bearing a medicine cup and I signaled for him to leave. This was not the time for an interruption. 'What do you want to do over the next 10 years?' I continued.

'Live with my wife, quietly. She is so beautiful. She has stayed with me, been my support and loved me. She is 65, but looks 20 years younger. People don't believe it seeing us together.'

'I'm sure she is so loving to you because of the way you are towards her.'

'Yes, I'm sure.'

'And your daughter too?'

'Yes, I role-modeled a caring father. She grew up straight and strong. She went to college and has a wonderful life so far. '

'The kind of life you weren't allowed to have.'

'No, not at all.' Now he was crying. Tears were streaming down his cheeks, flowing down beneath his hand that was covering his eyes.

This feels scary for me. At the edge of a precipice, don't know where is this going. Perhaps I'll just be quiet for a while. After what felt a long time, he commented:

'Now all I want is for my grandchildren to grow up. Enjoy them.'

I wonder if I can do it. Should I take the plunge? I don't want to make a fool of myself. But the timing feels right . . .

'Would you like a prayer?' I asked.

'I would love it!' he exclaimed.

Not being exactly sure what would emerge, I took his hand and leaned forward towards him as he covered his eyes with his other hand.

Dear God. Your son is in a lot of emotional pain. He had a terrible childhood. He was trapped in a family with no love, no caring, no support. No one he could trust to be there for him. It has affected him his whole life. Even now.

We thank you for all the blessings you have sent him: a wonderful wife, someone who has recognized his loving sensitive side, and returned his love and support in turn. We thank You, too, for his daughter and grandchildren, people who have, and will continue to, benefit from his love. We ask that he recover from surgery and have many more years to share with his family. We ask, not only for healing of this hole in his body, but also for healing of this hole in his soul.

Blessed is the Source of Life that accompanies and supports us in our journey.

Amen

'Yes, like a hole in the soul. Thank you Rabbi.' He was sobbing now. 'Thank you.'

We sat quietly for a moment, me still holding his hand, lightly.

'Thank you,' he said, once again.

'Rabbi. You know I have never ever shared this with anyone. My whole life I've never cried.'

I decided not to correct him. Somehow, it was important that he see me in the role of rabbi. Rising to leave, I thanked him for telling me his story.

'Thank *you*, Rabbi,' he responded in return.

As I walked out, I saw he was still lying with his hands covering his eyes.

I paused just outside his room. I felt quite shaken by this encounter not only by my impact on Joe, but also his impact on me.

That's when I overheard him say, 'At least one person understands. Thank God, one person knows.'

Same patient, same day, but a hugely different listening experience! I felt profoundly moved, and this supports the point that healing is never one-sided. I relieved his isolation, and in a lesser way he relieved mine. Far from being simple, this had been a complex active listening process that required my full attention with regards to content, timing and response.

- How much personal information was I to share? Too little prevented rapport. Too much crossed boundaries.
- What clues were being sent my way?

He seemed eager to speak when he immediately dispensed with the headphones. He was very friendly and chatty. May just be his personality but he seemed almost too forthcoming. Was there something beneath the surface?

He expressed an introject. (Did you notice it?) He said, 'I can't complain.' I challenged his introject when I asked, 'Why can't you complain?' In other words, where did you learn you can't complain? Which authority figure instilled this in you? Then he said, 'It was God's will.' Well, there is no higher authority than this! As God's perceived representative, I supported his complaint and validated his suffering. This was healing for him.

When he tried to shift the conversation, I sensed that this was making him uncomfortable and therefore there was more that needed to emerge.

- When was speech helpful? When was silence better?
- What words reflected back allowed him to feel heard, understood, supported yet not parroted? I decided to mirror his words in the form of a prayer.
- What metaphor created a helpful image? In this case, the wound in Joseph's psyche seemed greater than the wound in his body. He resonated with this by repeating the quote.
- He projected the role of rabbi onto me. Was I to allow him to do so or was I to correct him? In this case I chose to let it slip since it must have served a purpose.

Conclusion

There are very few fortunate people whose personalities and life experience allow them to be naturally empathetic, deep listeners. Then there are the rest of us. We require training to use our intellect to help guide us as we listen. This makes our listening no less moving as in the case of my listening to Joseph.

The most important part of this encounter was non-verbal. I centered and supported myself prior to entering the room. Somehow my body language, tone of voice, words, title, signaled to him that I could be trusted and was interested in listening. As a result, he opened up to me in a way that he hadn't to others.

This listening encounter demonstrates the vast difference in complexity in listening to the patient versus listening to the disease.

On a practical level, it is well known that patients with chronic back pain have a high incidence of depression. Back pain not only disables physically, it also adversely impacts emotional and spiritual well-being. Boredom, absence of meaning, loss of income, frustration and despondency might cause some to smoke and eat more. Prolonged rest leads to muscle atrophy and weight gain. Even 'successful' surgery may be followed by further disability as other joints and disk spaces are affected.

Listening in this situation enables the clinician to hear the patient and offer the support needed to lessen the risk of chronic disability.

Practice points

- You may be neither a chaplain nor a therapist, yet as a healthcare professional you occupy a place of privilege in society. You are present at exquisitely intimate moments in the lives and deaths of people. There is a spectrum of communication that ranges from superficial to very deep. The times you listen with focused attention will be for you, as it has been for me, the most magical and memorable encounters of your professional life.
- Some of the time, simple gathering of facts will do. Increasingly you will find as you keep your ears cocked for clues that there is much more going on than appears at first glance. If necessary, pause to listen more deeply. Patients intuit your willingness to listen and will share private information. It will always be significant, and patients will rarely abuse your time. Almost invariably, this results in improvement in medical care.
- It is not easy to pray spontaneously with a patient. Even chaplains with many years of experience stumble. On the occasion that you may be asked to do so, reflecting back what you have heard in the form of a prayer will create a powerful and empowering experience for your patient.
- Once you successfully master the complexities of using listening as a healing technique you will encounter an entirely new dimension of practice.

7

But listening is so passive

Patience is not passive; on the contrary it is active;
it is concentrated strength.
Edward G. Bulwer-Lytton, 1803–73

Introject: the role of the physician is to be active, and listening seems so passive.

We have seen that patients are frequently interrupted in their opening statements and given little time to express themselves fully thereafter. Lack of time may explain the need to interrupt, but what if this isn't the only reason? What if there is a deeper, less obvious reason, namely the perception that listening is passive?

The rigorous process of becoming a physician effectively weeds out passive students. If this was not enough, many emerge from residency training deeply in debt and needing to catch up on lost income. Once in practice, physicians are not compensated for being passive. Physicians *take* a history, *perform* an examination, *review* laboratory results, *order* treatment, and *write* prescriptions – i.e., are active.

Listening, on the other hand, requires mostly silence – and this *feels* very passive. It seems as if all the activity is in the speaker's corner.

And of course, this is grossly misleading.

Yes, the speaker is actively speaking. But, the speaker is also listening to his own voice; hearing his thoughts expressed aloud perhaps for the first time, and this may well alter his understanding of his issues. Not only is the speaker listening to his own voice, he is also actively listening to the body language and verbal responses of the listener to see how his words are being received.

The listener, as we have seen in the last chapter, is also being active. Depending on the nature of the encounter, the listener:

- attends to the boundaries of the interaction
- clears her mind of distractions so as to be fully present in the here and now

- observes who is in the room, what is at the bedside, what is the patient doing, how is he dressed, what is his demeanor
- hears with focused yet relaxed attention
- utilizes all her senses, including vision, to search for non-verbal cues
- listens for hints of the emotions behind the words
- checks her own emotions to assess the impact of the other's words
- evaluates the communication in the light of her professional knowledge
- consciously seeks the story behind the story, since the presenting issue is often not the real issue; what is *not* articulated is frequently more important than what *is*
- reflects back empathy and understanding, being careful not to instinctively judge or offer premature suggestions
- is attentive to her own body language.

The reality is that there is nothing about listening that is passive. In the following encounter I used my eyes when listening. What my eyes heard transformed my understanding of the patient and led to a breakthrough in his management. And, it also led to a fight:

Despite my best efforts, Bob kept returning. If it was not his irritable bowel syndrome, it was his tension headaches or hyperventilation syndrome that resulted in him having episodes of full-blown panic attacks.

Standard history taking helped little. 'Nothing especially wrong Doc. Wife and kids are fine ... I own my own house ... the mortgage has to get paid ... job is good ... lots of responsibility being supervisor and keeping the shirt factory running smooth. I always have to be on my guard. I worry a lot about money. I wish my wife would work. Instead she hops from job to job – without ever taking her work too seriously. Now she's unemployed again. I don't think I'm unusual. I guess everybody has some things that bother them, not so?'

The medicines I prescribed for his headaches, diarrhea, cramps, dizzy spells helped a little, but still his symptoms persisted. As for psychotherapy, Bob did not feel he needed it.

One might imagine that Bob, age 37, would look haggard and tense. In fact, he was dapperly dressed, mostly smiling and pleasant; disarmingly so.

One day we had a breakthrough. It occurred after I asked him about his family. 'Funny you should ask,' he responded. 'I just had a run in with the wife. Women! I came home from work, gave her my coat to hang up in the closet, same as always, and she wouldn't! So I told her off and we had the usual row about her not working, and all I wanted from her was to hang up my coat! Was I being unreasonable?'

I wasn't paying as much attention to his words as I was to his body language. Here he was describing an argument and he was smiling and his posture seemed relaxed. Words and body language did not match. When he should have been tense and upset he seemed totally in control – so much so that he had no healthy release of tension, anger, and frustration. No wonder he had all those stress-related physical symptoms.

I could explain this to him, but it was unlikely to be helpful. Perhaps if he experienced an absence of control it would raise his awareness.

'Bob, do you think you are ready to try some therapy?'
'What exactly do you mean by therapy?'
'Well, more than just talking *about* your issues. Do you trust me?'
He said, 'yes,' so I threw the pillow at him.
'WA WHATCHA DO THAT FOR!' Bob exclaimed.

I had just walked over to the exam table and thrown a pillow at him very lightly, still it caught him by surprise.
'Toss it back to me,' I instructed.
'No, I can't do that – you're the doctor!' he spluttered.

I took the pillow from him – he was still staring at it in bewilderment – then threw it back to him again, this time more forcefully. This added to his confusion.
'What's this all about, why are you throwing the pillow?' he asked.
'Come on Bob, throw it back. You ever been in a pillow fight?'

Ever so lightly, he flipped it back. Now I hurled it towards him saying as I did so, 'You can do better than that.'

This time the pillow sailed past me and struck the wall, narrowly missing a photograph. Back and forth the pillow flew until a few feathers started to float ominously in the air. The paper pillowcase was in shreds. Time to end. I caught the pillow and returned it to its permanent spot on the exam table. Bob was panting. I noticed his tie was crooked. Even his hair was a little disheveled. He wore this slightly puzzled grin.
'How do you feel, Bob?'
'I feel great, Doc. What happened. What did you do?'

Barely suppressing a smile I countered with, 'This, Bob, was the therapy I offered you.'

Bob brushed his hair and rearranged his tie while I straightened the photograph. He now had a very different expression. Gone was the half smile. He appeared focused and attentive.
'How you doing?' I asked.
'I'm fine.'
'Surprised huh?'
'Yes, but I really feel much better, much looser.'

'It's been a while since you felt out of control like this?'

'Yes, But it was fun.'

'It's been a while since you had fun?'

'I always mean to take the boys rollerblading or fishing. Somehow I never find the time anymore. I always have so many responsibilities.'

'What feels more important to you are your responsibilities.'

'Right.'

'Keeping everything under control?'

'Yes. That's always been important to me. Not have any problems.'

'Must be a big strain huh?'

'It is.' He thought for a moment. 'So what you are suggesting is that maybe it would be better for me to loosen up, let go of control a bit. Not be under so much strain.'

'It makes sense. Any thoughts how you might do it?'

Bob thought for a while then, 'It might help for me to do the opposite of what I had always done. If I back off, perhaps Mary will pick up the slack.'

'You mean share some of your responsibility?'

'I never thought of it that way before.'

Bob made changes to his life and gradually his symptoms abated and his visits, to my delight, became less frequent.

On his last visit, he seemed rather proud of himself.

'Came home from work today Doc,' he said. 'My wife was there as usual, sitting reading on the sofa. She looked up as I entered the house and got up to take my coat. I had my hands behind my back, and as she approached me I whipped out the bunch of flowers I'd hidden. She was so surprised she actually started to cry! We kissed, then we spoke for an hour – not argued. You know this is the first time we'd spoken like this in years.' As he walked out through the door he shook his head and chuckled. 'I can't believe my doctor threw a pillow at me.'

Over the years, I had seen Bob many times and listened to his symptoms. When I finally listened to *him* rather than his symptoms, using all my senses, then things became clear.

Intellectual understanding would not help him. I needed to communicate to Bob in a non-verbal way that he was in a chronic state of control so that he could feel this in his body. I chose to raise his awareness of this by using a technique that would distract him from thinking, and would allow him to experience the opposite of control.

Those interested in compassion describe *compassionate listening*; others interested in spirituality describe *holy listening*; still others describe *active* _listening_. Such qualifiers are redundant. When listening skillfully, compassion, holiness, and active response emerge spontaneously without any prior agenda.

Practice points

- View the opening statement as a very specific part of the medical encounter, one which you consciously do not interrupt.
- Remind yourself that the act of _not_ interrupting is being active.
- Pause before you enter the room. Center yourself, become grounded and suspend your forward momentum. When you enter the room use your eyes. After your greeting, allow the story to unfold.
- Rather than just using verbal responses try occasionally to respond with silence, or the touch of a hand, or a nod of the head.
- Frequently words are just window-dressing and there is much going on behind the scenes. To really hear what is being communicated, pay attention to body language, choice of words, tone of voice, and really become aware of the emotions and story that lie behind the story. For example you may hear anger, but beneath anger is often shame or sadness, or feelings of isolation or rejection. Remember that unlike physical complaints, the presenting emotional issue is rarely the main issue.
- Silence on your part is a powerful technique that helps flush out hidden emotions. Stay with silence a little longer than may feel comfortable. See what emerges. This requires active suppression of your urge to speak.
- Don't be diverted by semantics. The term _active listening_ describes the activity of careful listening without judgment and confirming with the speaker that what is being communicated is being accurately understood. It naturally follows that if this is labeled active, then regular listening must be passive otherwise why qualify it? It may be best to avoid the term _active listening_ and instead view all careful, responsive listening as active.

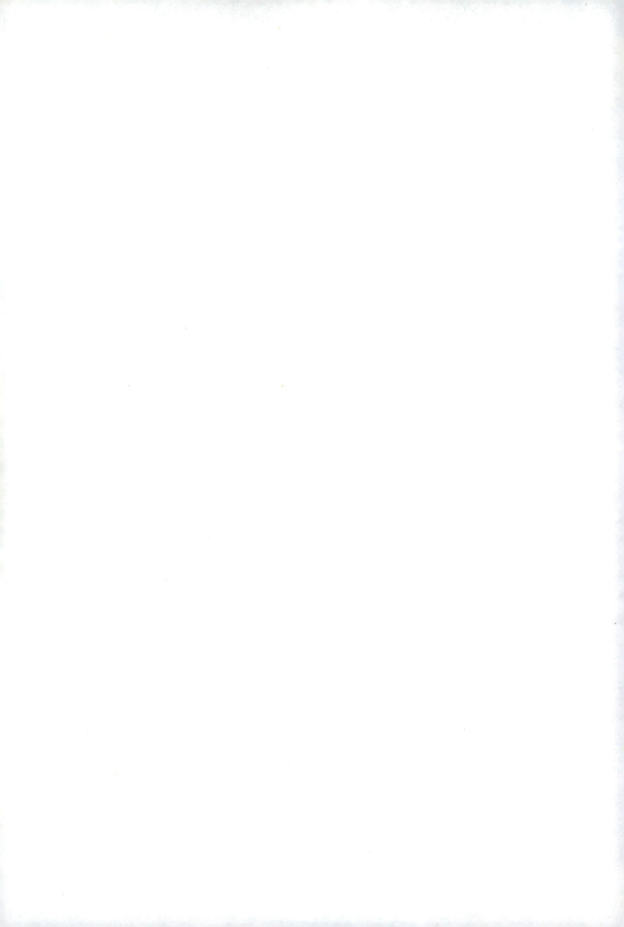

8

But listening leaves me without control

'You are very nice, but you *will* change.'
Patient to medical student

Introject: physicians should always be in control and listening to a patient's opening statement results in an uncomfortable role reversal, hence it is appropriate to interrupt and modify the course of the narrative.

Beyond the issue of time, pressure, and the need to be active, there is also the question of who is in control of the dialogue. It is tempting to think that the introject, *the patient should be passive and hand over total control*, begins with the first patient ... a corpse in the anatomy dissection room. No one is more passive and helpless than a dead body, and here the lowly student has absolute control. This is the ideal 'good' patient, one that does not fuss, speak, or demand attention.

Later, the student encounters his first live patient and is now hesitant, uncertain, vulnerable, empathetic, and often experienced as being very nice – hence the patient's comment, 'You are very nice, but you *will* change.'

The internship is a period of transition and stress in which time the student is expected to toughen up and become a competent physician. Mood disturbances increase and empathetic concern for patients decreases.[1]

While the intern is expected to be busy as never before, the patient, regardless of power and status outside, is expected to be a passive recipient of care with a life that now centers around the BED. Another shift in power and control has occurred.

Robbie E. Davis-Floyd writes of the contemporary ritual of childbirth in which the mother-to-be is treated as a birthing machine. She describes the ritual as involving induction of helplessness onto the patient from the moment she enters the hospital and is plopped onto the wheelchair. From then on, the system takes over, 'The open and exposing hospital gown, the ID bracelet, the intravenous fluid, the bed in which she is placed – all these convey to the laboring woman that she is dependent on the institution.'[2]

The patient, helpless and exposed in a flimsy gown lying on her back on an examination table, may experience the physician as the epitome of power and control.

One day, working as a chaplain, I was sitting at the bedside of a patient and listening to her story when a young resident entered the room, walked straight to the bedside and leaned over slightly to speak to her. At first I was miffed by the interruption and abuse of power, but then I noticed something. Because I was seated, my line of vision was directed straight to her waist, and attached to her belt were three beepers. Poor woman, I thought, one beeper is bad enough, but to be shackled to three beepers at the beck and call of anyone who called ... The illusion of power just melted away.

While physicians own a disproportionate amount of authority and power in the doctor–patient relationship, for most, this power does not spill over to their general professional and personal lives.

In the Kaiser survey of physicians conducted in 2001, 74% were dissatisfied with the amount of time they were forced to spend on administrative duties; 56% were unhappy with the time left for outside interests, family, and friends; and 54% were dissatisfied with the level of autonomy in clinical decisions.[3]

In the Women Physicians' Health Study conducted in 1999, it was found that work control was the factor most strongly correlated with career satisfaction.[4]

In the CTS Physician Survey conducted on primary care and specialist physicians 1997–2001, the strongest and most consistent predictors of change in satisfaction were changes in measures of clinical autonomy.[5]

All these surveys point to a lack of empowerment in practice and in lifestyle. Since, increasingly, physicians have limited autonomy and control over their own lives, where is this control displaced? Frequently over patients and those below them in the healthcare hierarchy as the following illustrates:

One study challenged the validity of restricting visitors' access to ICU patients except at 'rigidly specified times or with the doled-out permission of the ICU staff.' The authors invited several hospitals to liberalize visiting hours in ICUs and to evaluate the consequences. The authors pointedly noted, 'The mere proposal of this more liberal policy generated considerable resistance among nurses and physicians.' The fears of the healthcare professionals were that this new policy would stress patients, personnel, and visitors. This did not materialize. ...

The authors concluded, 'It is important that patients be able to decide who can visit them and when ...' and, 'Despite the resistance the results were uniformly positive for all concerned.'[6]

In the study quoted above, the authors had proposed something quite radical, i.e., that the locus of power be shifted to patients who could then decide who they wished to have visit them and when.

A basic principle of trauma management is the restoration of a sense of power and control to the victims. Patients in intensive care units are traumatized and, as the study showed, their having a say in who can visit them and when lessened their stress rather than increased it.

Conclusion

Many patients, particularly ones with chronic illness, prefer to have an active role in the management of their disease process and overall health. They will frequently utilize their physicians primarily as consultants.

Physicians, too, want more autonomy and control, and their reclaiming genuine personal and professional empowerment may lessen the need for power to be displaced over others, in particular, patients.

Hopefully the day will arrive when physicians no longer claim: 'We care for our patients.' Instead, the mantra will be: 'We care for ourselves AND we conscientiously partner our patients in their care of themselves.'

This will be reflected in communication style in which patients will be empowered to speak without feeling pressured, and in which there is more inquiry, invitation to raise issues of concern, and respectful listening.

Practice points

Reclaim your own empowerment in areas that matter to you

Create white space in your life

It is almost impossible to experience power if you are overwhelmed by the *too much to do, too little time* phenomenon. Unless you achieve some healthy relationship with time and creation of white space in your life, you will find yourself in a constant uphill battle against lack of time. Use organization, simplicity, streamlining, and collaboration to create space. Consider utilizing a healthcare consultant to aid you in this.

Adolescent patients routinely require physical examinations for sport, driving licenses, jobs, school, etc. Good screening involved asking about high-risk issues such as driving safety, sexually transmitted diseases, depression, suicidal ideation, substance abuse, diet, family dynamics, and relationships. Faced with this daunting and time-consuming task several times a day, I invested a number of hours designing a highly comprehensive standardized self-administered questionnaire for teenagers that would cover all physicals – driver, sport, work, etc. I invested time in training my employees to verify immunizations, check vision, hearing, and vital signs. As a result, my routine adolescent physical examinations became more thorough than most, yet only took up a few minutes of my time.

Hold onto the power you have

How often do I hear, 'I can't ... if only ... I must ... managed care won't let me ... I'd like to but ... etc.'

A patient with innumerable nevi and a family history of malignant melanoma asked to be seen by a dermatologist. Though nothing seemed suspicious, I agreed to the referral both to reassure her and not to leave myself open to liability should a melanoma develop.

A few weeks later, the medical director of her HMO called me and asked if I would photograph her nevi and mail the photographs to him. He would make the determination if referral was necessary.

Rather than to acquiesce to this inappropriate use of power, I took a deep breath, leaned back in my armchair, stared at my favorite photograph – a 2 feet by 3 feet enlargement of a nature scene I had taken on one of my vacations, and replied, 'I never studied medical photography, but if you wish to photograph her yourself (involving a drive of 90 miles each way) please come to town and do so. You can even use my office.'

'I'll approve her this time,' he growled, 'but next time I want photos.'

Just as well he could not see my grin.

Collaborate with your colleagues to reclaim power

Isolation is disempowering. Little is accomplished as a solitary voice. Work with your colleagues towards shifting the center of power away from bureaucrats, legislators, and lawyers. Once again, in the short term it involves the use of your time. In the long run this becomes a highly profitable investment.

When our county medical society ignored my request for services I resigned and created the Physician Interactive Group (PIG). This was an organization of 20 family physicians that met monthly at a restaurant over dinner while we socialized and shared topics of common interest. We also designed forms and material that we could use in our respective offices to save ourselves time and increase efficiency. As the president of this little group, I had to fend off hospital administrators, specialists, bank managers, and others who were eager to speak with us. The medical society scrambled to upgrade its services, and I eventually restored my membership.

Share empowerment with patients in areas that matter to them

Illness and engagement with the healthcare system strip power away from the typical patient. The entire environment is unfamiliar, intimidating, and frightening, especially as patients are dependent on others for guidance and help. One reason that billions of dollars are spent on over-the-counter, alternative therapies, and 'health' products is that these empower patients to do something for themselves rather than feel passive and helpless. Between 1990 and 1997, the US population increased its use of herbal medicines by 380%, and total out-of-pocket expenditures in 1997 were $5.1 billion.[7]

Whenever possible, offer your patients choices and invite their participation in decision making. If you see a patient is significantly obese, don't simply warn of the consequences and prescribe a diet. Ask your patient how he or she feels about it. Ask how you can be of help. Shift responsibility to your patient rather than retaining it all for yourself.

The opening statement is a specific and unusual situation in which the patient can take the conversation in any direction that feels important — that is until you interrupt and reclaim control. Regard this statement as special and see where it goes.

When doing an elective procedure clarify your patient's wishes. A unique situation is childbirth. This is not just a medical event; it is a major lifecycle event for the patient and her family. Have the patient create a *wish list* regarding the delivery – who she wants at delivery, what type of analgesia, how she wants the newborn handled, etc. Many of these wishes are highly important to the mother. Review the list with her, and add the wishes that are important to you or gently modify hers if they are impractical. This way you share power, establish dialogue, and create a partnership.

References

1   Bellini L, Baime M, Shea J (2002) Variation of mood and empathy during internship. *JAMA*. **287**: 3143–6.

2   Grimes RL (1996) *Readings in Ritual Studies*, pp. 146–58. Prentice-Hall, New Jersey.

3   Kaiser Family Foundation (2002) National Survey of Physicians. (Conducted March–October 2001.) www.kff.org/kaiserpolls/3223-index.cfm

4   Frank E, McMurray J, Linzer M *et al.* (1999) Career satisfaction of US women physicians. *Arch Intern Med*. **159**: 1417–26.

5   Landon B, Reschovsky J, Blumenthal D (2003) Changes in career satisfaction among primary care and specialist physicians, 1997–2001. *JAMA*. **289**: 442–9.

6   Berwick DM, Kotagal M (2004) Restricted visiting hours in ICUs: time to change. *JAMA*. **292**: 736–7.

7   Ernst E (2005) How to judge a herbal remedy. *OBG Management*. **17**: 28–35.

9

But there's no room for emotions inside this white coat

'... a single expression of sorrow or regret – one indication that it mattered to them even a fraction as much as it mattered to us – would almost have changed everything.'

A breast cancer patient on being given the news that bone-marrow transplants were ineffective

Introject: professionalism requires that physicians be objective. Since emotions tend to get in the way of good medical care and affect physician well-being, they need to be examined and controlled.

Emotions are challenging. These little beasts tend to show up at the most inconvenient time. We physicians pride ourselves on our scientific objectivity, and when these rascals emerge from their hiding place we are taught they need to be collared, examined, and then locked up so they won't interfere.

A journal article, 'The inner life of physicians and care of the seriously ill,'[1] opens up a Pandora's Box as it unbuttons that sterile veneer of objectivity, the white coat, and displays a host of emotions that may adversely affect both quality of care and physician well-being. The authors point out that physicians react to seriously ill patients with a variety of emotions which, if unexamined, can lead to 'physician distress, disengagement, burnout, and poor judgment.' The conclusion is reached that '... physicians should take an active role in identifying and *controlling* those emotions.'

At first glance this conclusion sounds so reasonable that the introject it expresses may easily be overlooked. After all, something needs to be done with emotions – one need only think of medical students who, left unchecked, may spill their emotions uncontrollably. For example:

- *Anxiety*. In an article entitled 'Don't discuss it: reconciling illness, dying, and death in a medical school anatomy laboratory,'[2] the author describes her study of communications in an anatomy dissection laboratory. She writes:

Particular attention is given to the history and maintenance of the medical faculty's tacit prohibition against discussion of their own and their students' attitudes and anxieties about illness, dying and death. She also makes note of what she describes as 'a conspiracy of silence between professors and students and between students and their fellow students.' Even today, when there tends to be a more enlightened approach of openness, students still often hide their discomfort behind cynicism and humor.

- *Compassion and grief.* In a 55-word narrative,[3] this student writes about her crisis — her fork in the road. *Do I remain compassionate and suffer? Or do I become desensitized and tough in which case I'll have lost my humanity.'*

> The Student's Dilemma: In the hospital's predawn stillness, she confided fears about surgery to me, the medical student. I tried to reassure her. They operated. Finding extensive metastases, they closed immediately. That evening, aching for her, I cried. 'Don't worry,' another student reassured me. 'It gets easier.' 'I hope not. If it does, I'll have lost my humanity.'

- *Excitement.* David, a medical student, loved clinical medicine and was uninhibited in the way he shared his excitement. His voice would carry across the open wards, 'Wowwww, did you guys feel this liver!' or 'Guys, you gotta come and see this!' Patients would turn ashen and I would cringe. Eventually, he learnt to be more tactful and controlled. Still, once in a while he would express himself with a low whistle. Fortunately David went on to become a psychiatrist.

Infants and children can be delightful (and embarrassingly honest) when they express their emotions spontaneously and openly. Then they learn to modulate their expressions in ways that are socially acceptable. Young adults who choose to become medical students are confronted by situations they have never before encountered, and one of their developmental tasks is to develop appropriate coping strategies to handle their emotions.

The faculty in the anatomy laboratory role-modeled silence as an appropriate way of dealing with emotions.

The distressed medical student used reassurance as a response to her patient's fear, and in turn received reassurance from her fellow student when she was distressed. Here reassurance was used to modulate or control the emotions of another — unsuccessfully, as it turns out.

David learned to filter and modify his exuberant expressions of excitement.

In none of these situations were emotions welcomed, listened to, accepted without judgment, validated, and supported. Instead they were suppressed or aborted with reassurance. In each case *control* was the method of choice in dealing with emotions.

For medical students, so much knowledge must be acquired in four short years that it is far more expedient to create an environment where the experience and expression of emotions is simply discouraged, than it is to incorporate programs that facilitate personal reflection and incorporation of emotions. Where such programs do exist, they are frequently inadequate.

One student wrote, 'We masked our emotions and curbed our imaginations in favor of scientific interest. It was a sink-or-swim introduction to shutting off our feelings.'[4]

There are many reasons why masking and suppressing emotions presents a problem.

- Many students have a history of serious trauma prior to entering medical school.[5] They inevitably encounter situations that retrigger their traumas and result in behavior that is not necessarily in the best interest of themselves and their patients. Processing their own emotions may be helpful in raising their awareness of issues and situations related to traumas that are troublesome to them.
- It takes energy to control emotions. Far from protecting against burnout (another myth), application of control over part of oneself as a coping tool is more likely to stimulate it. The use of control sets up a conflict between intellect and emotion, the one suppressing the other wishing to assert itself. This struggle drains energy, suppresses vitality, and is self-destructive.
- Emotional health is greatest when knowledge (intellect) and feeling (emotion) are cultivated and integrated rather than separated. Many people spend years in psychotherapy trying to accomplish this. The culture of medicine encourages the opposite. When intellect and emotion *support* each other, rather than control each other, the result is emotional health, harmony, and personal empowerment.
- Control of emotions cannot be totally selective. Suppression of 'negative emotions' is likely to cause suppression of joy and compassion as well. A full range of emotions is needed for healthy relationship and function.
- Far from being an inconvenience, emotions are essential for empathy, compassion, communication, and healing. When the practitioner listens to his or her emotions as valuable (albeit sometimes painful) messengers, they fade into the background. When they are ignored or suppressed they call out even louder, may inadvertently and unconsciously emerge, and then endanger the physician–patient and other relationships.[6]

- Many physicians already control their emotions by burying 'them' under work or medicating them with alcohol, drugs, workouts at the gym, and even stress reduction techniques. In a profession where medical mistakes trigger a great deal of anxiety, fear, guilt, and shame;[7] where a high level of stress is the norm for other reasons as well; it is tempting to speculate that this control, stoicism, and silence are factors that result in a physician suicide rate that is significantly higher than that of the general population.[8]

- The more comfortable a physician is with her own emotions, the more she is able to tolerate and even welcome the emotions of others. In the movies of the 1950s, when the heroine hears bad news and is shocked, the hero typically rushes to pour her a shot of whiskey. 'Here, drink this, it will help,' he says. Medical practice is much like this, with physicians being trained to rush for tranquilizers and antidepressants in order to suppress the fears and tears of patients.

- When emotions are suppressed, then they need to be replaced by something. An authentic smile becomes a forced smile. Genuine empathy may be replaced by empathy that is acted[9] or even worse by distance and stilted affect. Professionalism requires that conscious expression of empathy be part of the routine, yet when totally acted out, an expression of emotion can be exaggerated or inappropriate.

Jerry had a total knee replacement and in the immediate post-operative period suffered excruciating pain. His orthopedic surgeon, however, would radiate complete cheer and well-being as he 'waltzed' into the room. 'If I talked about my pain or asked a question, he would instantly lose his broad smile and take a step back as if he wanted to escape from the room,' Jerry reported.

- When emotions are suppressed, the subtle ones that lurk in the shadows of the loudest are also never given the opportunity to see the light of day. All are uniformly suppressed, and tend to seep out as laments, cynicism, anger, irritability.

- Ironically, the suppression of emotions may be counterproductive. There is always the risk that pent-up emotions may burst out, like a dam break. This may occur at highly inappropriate moments and may well interfere with professionalism.

Despite this, the article 'The inner life of physicians and care of the seriously ill'[1] perpetuates the myth that feelings are best examined and controlled.

In the following example, the resident's underlying problem was one of too much control, not too little. Times are slowly changing in medical schools with the introduction of creative programs such as narrative medicine, medical humanities, etc. Still, it comes too late for some, and those pesky critters that emotions are, eventually find a way of escaping from their cage ...

The patient was a sorry sight. Overweight, gray unkempt hair, disheveled shabby clothes, she sat with shoulders slumped. Leaning over her was the handsome, well-groomed resident, his red necktie neatly knotted and pale blue shirt crisply starched. I could not hear him through the one-way glass, but could see him aggressively wagging a finger at her. 'What's up, you seem angry,' I commented when he emerged from the examination room.

'She hasn't lost weight, she smokes, her blood glucose is high and she's dirty. She's a pig and she's wasting my time.'

Startled by his angry outburst and somewhat appalled by his attitude I suggested we meet later to review this incident. Later, rather than telling him to control his temper, I thought I would try to learn more about him.

'What made you decide to do medicine as a profession?' I asked.

'It was my parents' idea. I always wanted to be a professional basketball player; I was good at it too.'

'You had to set aside your dreams to fulfill theirs?' I responded.

'Yes, exactly, and I hated doing it. Every day was a struggle for me. It doesn't get easier and now I don't even have time for an occasional game.'

'How did you manage to succeed when you hated it so much?' I asked.

'Through determination, discipline, and hard work. I don't dwell on it, though. Anybody can do anything if they try hard enough.'

Even a poor fat, elderly woman with diabetes I thought.

Ted had learnt his lesson well. He used control to suppress the anger that was eating away at him. No doubt he had other emotions, perhaps guilt at feeling so angry, shame at failure, frustration, sadness, etc. He needed a safe supportive environment (i.e., therapist's office) for venting and processing his feelings. Instead, he focused on being a good physician, and his emotions built up and were projected safely onto hapless patients.

It is conceivable that, later on in his career, Ted may well become a 'disruptive' physician. A less-disciplined individual or one with an addictive personality might well end up abusing drugs or alcohol as well.

Contrary to the prevailing introject that personal well-being and patient care are best served by students and physicians examining and controlling their emotions, authentic communication requires access to a full range of emotions. An alternative approach is to set aside times for introspection; to welcome emotions rather than to distance from them; to approach emotions with curiosity rather than judgment; to integrate them as an aspect of oneself rather than to isolate and attempt to control them.

Practice points

Claim ownership of your emotions

The more your emotions become yours, the less likely you are to project them onto others. You can only know how you feel; you cannot assume to know how others feel. Take a few minutes to ask yourself the following questions.

- Do I welcome my feelings as an aid to my relationship with myself and others or do I experience them as getting in the way?
- Do I judge and label my emotions as being good or bad, positive or negative?
- Do I only have an inner critic or do I also have an inner supporter?
- Do I acknowledge the need for compassion for myself, or do I displace it onto others?

Create space in your life for emotions to emerge and be acknowledged

The more rushed you are, the more you connect with your most superficial emotions – the ones that are loudest and most immediately accessible. It is difficult to examine emotions that are deeper and less obvious. Consider studying a technique such as Focusing that helps you access these.[10] As emotions are listened to, they reveal themselves like layers of onion being peeled and eventually become incorporated to be replaced by tranquility.

Join mental health professionals in attending workshops and training programs that enable you to participate in reflective educational experiences.

Group discussion may be of great value in raising your awareness of personal issues needing attention. Possibilities include Balint, creative writing, narrative, support, or supervision groups.

Ventilate both alone and with colleagues or friends

David Lee writes about the ritual of the morning tea break at which time nurses come together to have tea and 'to get things off their chest by laughing, yelling, and talking loudly about their problems at work and most importantly, gaining each other's support and regaining their internal balance.'[11]

Do not hesitate to seek help if you feel chronically emotionally overwhelmed or drained

It may be the best investment you will ever make. By all means share your feelings with close friends and colleagues, but not at the expense of seeing a professional therapist or mentor when necessary. Many journal articles suggest consulting a 'trusted colleague' if stressed. The result is likely to be comforting rather than therapeutic, since expressions of extreme grief or anger need the safety of an extremely intimate or appropriate professional relationship.

Do be concerned if you feel numbed and without emotion. You may be depressed or suffering from burnout.

Learn to use your emotions

Should an emotion emerge for you while you are with a patient, take note of it and decide whether to use it in your communication with your patient, e.g., 'As I hear your story about your mother, I feel sad. Yet I notice you are smiling. Why am I holding the sadness yet you seem unperturbed?'

If your emotion is a distraction, practice 'parking' it, i.e., acknowledging the emotion, then setting it aside with a clear understanding that you will return to it later.

Know your degree of emotional responsiveness

People vary in their degree of emotional responsiveness. The same trigger that causes a huge reaction in one individual may cause barely a ripple in another. A child falls and scrapes a knee. One mother may respond, 'Oh my poor baby, how could such a thing have happened to you? Are you okay?'

while another, barely concerned, responds 'It's just a scraped knee, you'll be fine.' This trait is easy revealed in graphoanalysis where the degree of slant of the upstroke relates to the degree of responsiveness. Responsiveness can be compared to the ripples in a pond when a stone is tossed in. Some ponds will ripple more – the shallower the pond, the greater the ripples. Experience, certain spiritual and mindfulness practices help 'deepen the pond' so that one can react with more equanimity.

Professionalism requires a healthy appreciation that, unlike in the example of David the exuberant student, the experience of an emotion and the expression of it must be separated. Now, experiencing emotional response, bringing it to conscious awareness and expressing it become three distinct phases.

Imagine the following scenario. An ill child is brought by his mother to the clinic. He can be seen by either of three physicians.

1   Dr A's internal reaction is low on the response curve. He comes across as unfeeling and uncaring.
2   Dr B's reaction is intermediate on the response curve. He has however introjected that the appropriate professional approach is to be calm, unemotional, and reassuring. He too comes across as being somewhat unfeeling.
3   Dr C's reaction is high on the response curve. He lost a patient once with the same condition. He panics the mother by his reaction since he seems so concerned.

Good practice requires that each factors in his degree of emotional responsiveness, adjusting his response, tone of voice and words accordingly. This way, intellect partners but does not control emotion.

Do not suppress the emotions of others with premature reassurance or words of comfort

The best response is affirmation, silence, or the expression of an emotion that resides in you, if appropriate. Instead of reassuring her patient the student in the 55-word story cited earlier could have responded with, 'This is such a frightening situation,' or 'I feel sad that you have to go through this experience,' or non-verbally with silence and a nodding of her head. She might also ask the patient, 'This is such an awful time for you, what can I do that would be helpful?' A gentle touch, too, signals caring.

To the extent that you are comfortable with your emotions, you will feel comfortable being with the emotions of others and be able to accept them without yours getting in the way.

When trauma stories are being told remember that, 'recollection without affect almost invariably produces no results.'[11] In other words, go beyond accepting grief reactions from your patients; welcome them as an essential component of healing.

References

1   Meir D, Back A, Morrison R (2001) The inner life of physicians and care of the seriously ill. *JAMA*. **286**: 3007–14.

2   William JL (1992) Don't discuss it: reconciling illness, dying, and death in a medical school anatomy laboratory. *Fam Syst Med*. **10**: 65–78.

3   Christianson A (2002) The student's dilemma. *JAMA*. **288**: 931.

4   Sharkey F (1982) *A Parting Gift*. St. Martin's Press, New York.

5   Ambuel B, Butler D, Hamberger LK *et al*. (2003) Female and male students' exposure to violence: Impact on well being and perceived capacity to help battered women. *J Compend Fam Stud*. **34**: 113–35.

6   Novack D, Suchman A, Clarck W *et al*. (1997) Calibrating the physician personal awareness and effective patient care. *JAMA*. **278**: 502–9.

7   Wu A, McPhee S, Christensen J (1997) *Behavioral Medicine in Primary Care: A Practical Guide*, pp. 299–306. Appleton & Lange, Stamford, CT.

8   Center C, Davis M, Detre T (2003) Confronting depression and suicide in physicians: a consensus statement. *JAMA*. **289**: 3161–6.

9   Larson E, Yao X (2005) Clinical empathy as emotional labor in the patient–physician relationship. *JAMA*. **293**: 1100–6.

10   www.focusing.org (accessed 27 June 2005).

11   Lee D (2001) The morning tea break ritual: a case study. *Int J Nurs Pract*. **7**: 69–73.

10

What to listen for: *psychological medicine*

I Hate You Don't Leave Me
Book title

As a healthcare professional, being a good listener is not enough .... Recognizing, appreciating, and understanding what is being communicated helps to shape specific and appropriate responses that enable the speaker to feel heard and understood. It also enables the practitioner to diagnose potentially serious disorders that need urgent treatment.

An editorial in the *BMJ* refers to study and practice of psychological aspects of patient care as *psychological medicine*.[1] This article makes the point that: 'At least 25–30% of primary-care patients have coexisting depressive, anxiety, somatoform, or alcohol misuse disorders.'[2] Additionally it states, 'Although physical symptoms account for more than half of all visits to doctors, at least a third of these symptoms remain medically unexplained.'[3,4] It is reasonable to assume that psychological factors are responsible for a significant portion of these. De Gruy, too, makes the case that a major portion of mental healthcare is rendered in the primary care setting and always will be.[5]

Mental and physical healthcare are inextricable linked, and knowledge of psychological medicine is essential for the care of the whole patient. When the mental and emotional aspect is denied, then situations such as the following become all too common.

Susan, a physician herself, went into premature labor because her obstetrician failed to notice that she had a uterine septum. The baby with a gestational age of only 24 weeks suffered severe brain damage and died. Years later, Susan remains traumatized, angry, and distressed with the themes in her narrative containing:

- *fear* even terror, as she went into premature labor
- *shame* that her uterus was 'deficient', unable to carry a baby to full term
- *guilt* that she chose this doctor when she should have known better and did not listen to her intuition for fear of being labeled a problem patient
- *forgiveness* issues with her condemnation of herself for being less than perfect
- *anger* towards the physician for being incompetent and insensitive.

In the following few chapters, some frequently encountered specific emotional and mental health conditions will be explored. They include fear, psychiatric issues, trauma, shame, and suffering.

Fear

Fear is an almost universally encountered condition in the healthcare setting. An acronym of Fear is *Future Events Appearing Real* and naturally the worst outcome frequently dominates the imagination of someone encountering illness or facing surgery.

Jerome was agitated, even panicky.

'Why hasn't my surgeon been around? Why have they started an intravenous infusion?' he wondered. He seemed puzzled by his doctor's absence as he waited for the result of the culture. A positive result would mean 6 weeks of parenteral antibiotics and enforced rest. A negative result meant he could have a new prosthetic hip implant and be on his feet in a few days. As I listened, I heard confusion, frustration, and fear. The failure of his physicians to communicate a rational plan of action seemed inexplicable to him. Intuitively, I asked what his profession had been prior to retirement.

'I was a pilot in the harbor. I would board a ship and even in the thickest fog, I could place the ship within a foot of where it needed to be. The captain could trust me,' he said.

'Who is the captain of *your* ship?' I asked, and this elderly man burst into tears.

'No one it seems,' he replied.

'So what do you need to do?' I continued.

'Call the surgeon's office,' he replied. 'I am going to do just that.'

Ultimately, his worst fears were to prove groundless and he received a new hip.

It is not always possible to eliminate fear or guarantee results, but it is *always* possible to elicit concerns and offer reassurance when appropriate. In this era of depersonalized care, it is immensely comforting having the knowledge that one is in good hands, i.e., someone is piloting the ship.

Some people live their lives trapped in fear. One 22-year-old was so reticent and withdrawn she seemed to be almost developmentally disabled. One day she handed me a slip of paper. On it she had written:

I feel fear
It's right here
In my mind
All the time
Everywhere I go
Please say it isn't so
How do I cope
When all I do is mope
I feel like a freak
Seven days of the week
Please say there is a cure
So I won't feel like this any more

I shed a tear
For I live in fear
There is no real danger
But these feelings are getting stranger.

While in this situation fear was pathological, it is safe to assume that fear is present to some extent in almost all patients and their loved ones.

Mood disorders

Important as it is to listen empathetically, it is even more important not to miss a life-threatening treatable psychiatric condition.

Mood disorders are extremely prevalent. The Surgeon General's report states that, in one year, about 7% of Americans suffer from mood disorders. About one-half of those with a primary diagnosis of major depression also have an anxiety disorder. Mood disorders rank among the top ten causes of worldwide disability,[6] and depression is frequently encountered in all practice settings, particularly in the elderly.[7]

Even though depression is well studied and understood, it is still frequently missed by physicians. In one study, only 17% of patients classified as clinically anxious and only 6% of those classified as clinically depressed were perceived as such by their oncologists.[8]

In a telephone survey during 1997 and 1998, 1636 adults with a probably depressive or anxiety disorder were interviewed. Of these, 83% had seen a healthcare professional, with most seeing a primary care physician. Of this group, only 19% received appropriate treatment.[9]

In another survey, physicians responded positively to patient clues about their emotional state in only 38% of surgical cases and 21% in primary care settings.[10]

The seriousness of the situation cannot be overstated. Whereas only 5% of older patients who kill themselves have seen a mental health professional during the 3 months before death, 70% have seen their primary care physician in this time period, with up to 25% having seen their physician within one day.[11]

In a study of 1354 patients who died of suicide over a 9-year period in Ontario, Canada, it was found that one-half had visited a physician within the preceding week.[12]

The diagnosis and treatment of depression will not be covered here since there are many resources available for learning more about this common condition. The main point is to always keep the possibility of serious clinical depression and impending suicide in mind. Communication and healing support medical treatment but do not replace it.

Personality disorders

You are an internist. Across from you is an attractive, well-dressed, intelligent woman who says that she is pleased to be joining your practice, she has heard wonderful things about you, and she looks forward to being your patient for many years. You feel somewhat flattered by her attention and anticipate a long relationship.

Over the next few months she seems increasingly enamored by you and spreads the word to all her friends. You notice, however, that she often calls for appointments at the last minute. Sometimes she arrives late and demands to be seen right away. On several occasions she asks for prescriptions to be called in without her being seen at all. You have this nagging discomfort about her, but reassure yourself that she really values and appreciates you. One day you receive an angry note that she is furious with you and that you will not be seeing her again.

'What have I done?' you ask yourself.

Perhaps nothing, since she may have a Borderline Personality Disorder or Adaptation (BPD) and is reacting to some perceived slight or rejection. All physicians have had the experience of patients unexpectedly leave their practice, and this may explain some of these occurrences.

As is the case with depression, the incidence of BPD is surprisingly high,[13,14] and in a significant percentage of cases, the condition is undiagnosed, and the primary care physician is unaware of any emotional or psychiatric disorder.[15]

Personality disorders are disorders of the *self*. They are very challenging, deep-seated, early adaptations that are not readily amenable to therapy or transformation. 'Individuals with personality disorder tend to project onto others one of the roles in their old, incomplete, interpersonal drama; and then they frequently misinterpret the other's response, because they are only seeing it from the point of view of their own unmet needs.'[16] For the patient who left your practice, for example, you might not be simply a father figure. You *are* the father!

Dr Eleanor Greenberg describes a simple screening test for personality disorders. Clients are asked to quickly choose which experience from their partner is most important to them in their relationships – love, admiration, or safety.

Most people are challenged to come up with a single clear-cut answer, but in her experience 'The Borderline client almost always chooses love over admiration or safety; the Narcissistic client prefers admiration to almost anything else; and the Schizoid client must feel safe at all costs or he or she cannot stay emotionally present to reap the benefits of either love or admiration.'[16]

BPD individuals tend to be attracted to people who they hope will love and care for them. Their relationships are intense, short-lived, and replaced by anger and hostility. They have little impulse control, and may abuse food, drugs, and alcohol. Healthcare professionals may easily be drawn into a care-giving role, then find themselves walking on eggshells between giving them the closeness and special attention they need and being too close and triggering fear and rejection.

Narcissists have little self-esteem, and structure their lives around receiving admiration and support, or else they experience self-deprecating depression. They work hard at impressing others and when they receive criticism they feel shame and humiliation. They tend to be overachievers and may be grandiose. Narcissists will flatter their healthcare professionals because they need to feel they have the best. Should they fail to receive the mirroring that they crave, should the professional seem less than the best, e.g., make a mistake, they may lash out angrily with hatred.

Schizoid individuals place safety as their foreground. They are terrified of being overwhelmed and having their identities annihilated. They need plenty of interpersonal space or else they will flee.

In each case, the individual tends not to fully engage with others for who they are as people. Rather they are perceived as objects that satisfy their unmet needs.

Antisocial Personality Disorder is one in which individuals seem incapable of experiencing shame, expressing remorse, and learning from their mistakes. They tend to run into trouble with the legal system since they repeatedly break the rules of society or their working environment, e.g., the military. There is frequently substantial psychiatric co-morbidity, and nearly two-thirds develop a lifetime alcohol or drug-use disorder.[17] Many end up in prison.

There is no effective therapeutic intervention for individuals with Antisocial Personality Disorder. The other personality disorders or adaptations may benefit from long-term therapy given by highly trained psychotherapists or psychiatrists.

Practice points

- You cannot afford to miss clinical depression.[18] Fully familiarize yourself with the symptoms and signs of depression, and always inquire about suicidal ideation when you are dealing with a depressed individual. When in doubt, refer for expert evaluation.
- Use written narrative as a form of communication. Consider asking your patients with chronic conditions (e.g., my patient with chronic fear) to write a poem or a short narrative to describe their experience of their issue or experience. Have them email it to you so you can review it at your leisure.
- Personality disorders are very challenging. On the one hand you do want to avoid labeling individuals since there is a stigma attached to being 'a borderline' or 'a narcissist'; on the other hand there are very practical reasons why you need to recognize personality disorders. You cannot presume that being 'reasonable' results in everyone being on the same page. Mostly, it requires that you adjust your interpersonal boundaries.
  - *Borderline Personality Disorder* patients benefit from firm predictable boundaries in all respects, payment, appointments, follow up, etc. Do not be lulled into negotiating exceptions.

- *Schizoid* patients need to be approached more tentatively and given extra space physically and emotionally. It is important that you attend to seemingly small details in seating arrangement, privacy, etc., so they feel safe.
- *Narcissistic* patients are prone to having their egos deflate if they sense criticism or have their self-image tarnished. They need those associated with them to be the best, and should something occur to disappoint them, they may take it very personally. Focus on building trust. Do not attempt to change their opinions. It is not helpful attempting to create insight and personal awareness, at least initially.[19]

References

1   Kroenke K (2002) Psychological medicine. Integrating psychological care into general medical practice. *BMJ USA.* **2**: 429–30.

2   Ormed J, Von Korff M, Ustun T *et al.* (1994) Common mental disorders and disability across cultures: results from the WHO collaborative study on psychological problems in general health care. *JAMA.* **272**: 1741–8.

3   Kroenke K (2001) Studying symptoms: sampling and measurement issues. *Ann Intern Med.* **134**: 844–55.

4   Reid S, Wessely S, Crayford T (2001) Medically unexplained symptoms in frequent attendees of secondary health care: retrospective cohort study. *BMJ.* **322**: 1–4.

5   De Gruy F (1997) Mental health care in the primary care setting: a paradigm problem. *Fam Syst Health.* **15**: 3–23.

6   www.surgeongeneral.gov/library/mentalhealth/chapter4/sec3.html   (accessed 19 June 2005).

7   Meldon S, Emerman C, Shubert D *et al.* (1997) Depression in geriatric ED patients: prevalence and recognition. *Ann Emerg Med.* **30**: 141–5.

8   Newell S, Sanson-Fisher RW, Bonaventura A (1998) How well do medical oncologists' perceptions reflect their patients' reported physical and psychosocial problems? Data from a survey of five oncologists. *Cancer.* **83**: 1640.

9   Young AS, Klap R, Sherbourne C *et al.* (2001) The quality of care for depressive and anxiety disorders in the United States. *Arch Gen Psychiatry.* **58**: 55–61.

10   Levinson W, Gorawara-Bhat R, Lamb J (2000) A study of patient clues and physician responses in primary care and surgical settings. *JAMA.* **284**: 1021–7.

11   Glaser V (2000) Topics in geriatrics: effective approaches to depression in older patients. *Patient Care.* **17**: 65–80.

12 Juurlink DN, Hertmann N, Szaalai J *et al.* (2004) Medical illness and the risk of suicide in the elderly. *Arch Intern Med.* **164**: 1179–84.

13 Sansone R, Whitecar P, Meier B *et al.* (2001) The prevalence of borderline personality among primary care patients with chronic pain. *Gen Hosp Psychiatry.* **23**: 193–7.

14 Moran P, Jenkins R, Blizard R *et al.* (2000) The prevalence of personality disorder among UK primary care attenders. *Acta Psychiatr Scand.* **102**: 52–7.

15 Gross R, Olfson M, Gameroff M *et al.* (2000) Borderline personality disorder in primary care. *Arch Intern Med.* **162**: 53–60.

16 Greenberg E (1998) Love, Admiration, or Safety: a system of Gestalt diagnosis of borderline, narcissistic, and schizoid adaptations that focuses on what is figure for the client. The 6th European Conference of Gestalt Therapy, 1–4 October 1998, Palermo, Italy.

17 Black D (2001) Antisocial personality disorder: the forgotten patients of psychiatry. *Primary Psychiatry.* **8**: 30–81.

18 Simon G, VonKorff M (1995) Recognition, management, and outcomes of depression in primary care. *Arch Fam Med.* **4**: 95–6.

19 Greenberg E (1996) When insight hurts: Gestalt therapy and the narcissistically-vulnerable client. *Br Gestalt J.* **5**: 113–20.

11

What to listen for:
trauma

'Of course you have plenty of experience with trauma, you went to medical school didn't you?'

A friend

Many young people enter the healthcare professions hoping to be healers. Then they discover environments that tend to be more traumatizing than healing. Realization sets in early as this following correspondence indicates:

Dear Doctor,
We have started a Wednesday morning lecture series given by family physicians and invite you to participate. As a group we enjoy meeting and talking with those doctors that are in the trenches.

Sincerely,
Rodney Goodman
Chief Resident

Dear Rodney,
Of course I will be delighted to participate. I was taken by your use of the phrase 'in the trenches'. This term is commonly used to describe medical practice today and it points to the experience of medicine as a battlefield. Perhaps my discussion can center on this perspective and what can be done about it.

Looking forward to hearing from you,
Barry Bub MD

Of course I did not hear back from him. As a physician, to speak of one's psychological trauma issues risks labeling oneself as weak and inadequate:

One of my clients, an obstetrician, has participated in a weekend coverage group for years and was finding most days on call horrendously stressful. Her colleagues frequently bickered when they felt unfairly burdened by the others' patients, yet they had not once had a meeting to discuss their problems or ways of supporting one another in a difficult environment.

Sometimes an admission of trauma slips out unconsciously when a physician confesses, 'I am one of the walking wounded,' or 'I am a recovering physician,' or sends an email such as the one I received just today from a residency director:

> Here is what I have been dealing with lately – a patient who made a very detailed threat to come in the office with a gun and kill everyone, on top of the very unexpected death of a 5-year-old who was seen by two residents 1 day apart, plus an increase in malpractice costs of 150% – well you know, the list goes on and on …

As a family physician, I never considered that trauma was a significant aspect of my work. Only much later did I discover that the life of a typical physician includes a spectrum of trauma that varies from chronic stress punctuated by moments of fear to acute catastrophic fright:

> I was stunned, bewildered and disoriented. Surely this wasn't happening to me. I felt cornered like a trapped animal and just had to escape so I spent most of the day wandering around in a daze. It was like living a dream, no, more like a nightmare.

The victim of an accident, criminal assault or terrorist attack? A woman with a spontaneous abortion? A Vietnam veteran whose entire platoon had been killed in an ambush? A patient given a diagnosis of inoperable cancer? An elderly lady whose husband died suddenly?

It could have been any of these. Even though trauma comes in many forms, *the neurobiological and hormonal response it triggers in the victim is the same* regardless of etiology. In this case it was an obstetrician describing his reaction to hearing he was being sued for medical malpractice.[1]

When he told some of his colleagues that he was being sued they attempted to reassure him that this was a 'normal part of medical practice'. Then they went on with their lives.

Patients experience trauma that may be catastrophic as well. Here is a physician describing her experience as a patient:

> That hospital was my personal place in hell. I have been constantly haunted by painful and awful memories of those four days as I am sure I will be

every day for the rest of my life. My newborn child was dying and I had to fight my case at the ethics committee meeting to have his life-support terminated. My brain was dazed from shock, trauma, caesarian section surgery, and lack of sleep. My obstetrician did not even have had the presence of mind to ask the chaplain or someone else to be there as a support for us.

Unimaginable as it might seem, her physician never once acknowledged her trauma or offered her a single word of comfort. Instead, she reassured her patient not to worry specifically pointing out that 'the next one will be just fine' – this as her baby lay dying.

Her friends were empathetic but clearly impatient for her to move on, and when she returned to work after a month's absence, her colleagues dismayed her by treating her as if she had been on vacation.

As these examples illustrate, both physicians and patients are linked in the experience of being seriously traumatized, and being additionally traumatized when their traumas are not validated and treated appropriately.

In contrast to prevailing wisdom that trauma victims seek safety and support, physicians who make a medical mistake or are sued tend to withdraw shamed and isolated in an environment that does not tolerate mistake or failure. They may never have the opportunity to reconstruct their trauma stories, remember and mourn their losses, develop healing therapeutic relationships, and return to society and their profession empowered and in control of their safety – all basic requirements for recovery.

Physicians whose traumas are denied are hardly likely to be sensitive to the traumas of their patients. The culture of denial that pervades trauma issues in physicians applies to patients as well, in whom trauma conditions are frequently underdiagnosed and undertreated.[2]

Physicians who suffer from traumatic stress disorders may manifest behavioral problems such as withdrawal, disruptive behavior, workaholism, drug and alcohol abuse. Needless to say, they do not make good communicators since they have difficulty creating healthy relationships. This may well be a limiting factor to communication, and one that is not overcome by the simple teaching of 'communication competencies'.

When trauma is denied, it follows that healing is denied as well. Since trauma and healing are flip sides of the same coin, both become the stepchildren of medicine.

There is relatively little in the medical literature indicating that both healthcare professionals and patients when exposed to sudden severe trauma may experience Acute Stress Disorder (ASD) or Reaction (ASR) – reminiscent of victims of serious accident, assault, war, or terrorism.

Major trauma

Acute stress disorder

In ASD, 'The individual has experienced or witnessed or was confronted with an unusually traumatic event that has *both* of these elements:

1 the event involved *actual or threatened death* or *serious physical injury* to the individual or to others, *and*
2 the individual felt *intense fear, horror* or *helplessness.*'[3]

This is a reaction that lasts for a minimum of 2 days and a maximum of 4 weeks. Symptoms include numbness, amnesia, disorientation, detachment, avoidance, anxiety, hyperarousal, flashbacks, dreams, and distress. Sometimes symptoms continue beyond 4 weeks, and the condition is then labeled Post-Traumatic Stress Disorder (PTSD).

Post-traumatic stress disorder

This is a chronic pervasive anxiety disorder characterized by symptoms clustered around three main areas:

1 re-experiencing the trauma
2 numbing of responsiveness or avoidance of thoughts or acts related to the trauma
3 excess arousal.[4]

As a consequence, individuals with PTSD tend to have intrusive reliving of thoughts, feelings, images, flashbacks, dreams of the trauma with associated autonomic hyperarousal. They tend to organize their lives around avoiding these intrusions, and may use alcohol, drugs, work, or dissociation to suppress these symptoms. Hyper-reactivity occurs even to minor stimuli and they either over-react or freeze. All emotion turns to anger. Symptoms may become somatized.[5]

Is trauma being trivialized?

I really don't think so. Society has historically tended to deny violence and discredit victims whether they suffered from hysteria, shell shock or sexual and domestic violence. Despite all the wars of the 20th century, it required the Vietnam veterans' movement, in 1980, to stimulate the inclusion of PTSD into the *Diagnostic and Statistical Manual of Psychiatric Disorders*. It is not surprising, then, that trauma in medicine would be denied. Initially, the description of PTSD required that trauma be 'outside the range of usual human experience'.[6] Later, it was appreciated that traumas triggering PTSD were all too common, so this criterion was dropped.

Currently the definition still requires *threaten death or serious physical injury*. Some believe[7] that that this criterion should be broadened to include *threatened severe emotional or spiritual injury*, since this seems to be the case.

While the classic manifestation of severe trauma is the condition known as PTSD, there are other disorders of extreme stress that may lack some of the typical characteristics of a full-blown PTSD. Judith Lewis Herman writes in *Trauma and Recovery*, 'People subjected to prolonged, repeated trauma develop an insidious, progressive form of post-traumatic stress disorder that invades and erodes the personality.' She continues, 'Not surprisingly, the repetition of trauma amplifies all the hyperarousal symptoms of post-traumatic stress disorder.'[6] Chronic stress of this magnitude is not uncommon in medical practice or in severe life-threatening illness and affects professionals, patients, and their loved ones.

There are some references to the effects of severe trauma to physicians in the literature:

- Dr Ronald Hofeldt, a psychiatrist who is director of physician affairs for Physicians Insurance, described litigation stress as '... an acute stress reaction that over time becomes chronic, not unlike post-traumatic stress disorder. The acute stress corresponds with the initiation of the suit, but since a lawsuit proceeds in fits and starts over a period of years, the trauma continues, on and off, and creates chronic stress symptoms.'[8] Depositions, letters from attorneys, correspondence with hospital credential committees, and testimony in court – all are cues reminding the 'victim' of the incident and trigger hyperarousal effect and anxiety.
- Dr James Kennedy, in a letter to *JAMA*, stated that it is his belief that most physicians have PTSD which he attributes to toxic shame, 'During their training, physicians experience both physical (80–100-hour workweeks) and emotional (shaming by professors and supervising house staff) abuse. Once in practice, patient care "retriggers" the toxic fear, loneliness, pain, anger, and shame physicians experience in training. I believe these extreme feelings are related to PTSD.'[9]

Other major traumas for physicians

Suicide of a patient

This is perhaps the most distressing of all events for psychotherapists and psychiatrists as one article attests:

Their reactions may be roughly compared to that of combat soldiers ...' and 'Some of these six therapists experience an extreme level of shock; one developed what he described as post-traumatic stress syndrome after the surprising suicide of his patient ...'[10]

Medical mistakes

The accusation, perception, or discovery of a medical mistake is an event '... evoking intense emotions of shock, remorse, guilt, anger, and fear.'[11] Mistakes are all too frequent with the IOM report in 1991 suggesting that 44 000–98 000 patients die from medical error every year in the USA, with a much greater number being injured.[12] If only a small percentage of physicians are traumatized by having committed a serious error, the numbers would still be large.

Severe traumas for patients

Sudden and unexpected death of a loved one

The commonest cause of PTSD in the general public is reported to be the sudden and unexpected death of a loved one.[13] It is tempting to speculate that unrecognized and untreated PTSD may be one reason why insomnia and dependence on sedatives is so prevalent in elderly widows.

It is not uncommon for the primary care physician to be called by a son or daughter with, 'Father died suddenly, mother needs a sleeping pill' or 'Mother needs something to calm her so she is able to handle the funeral.' Mother may well have an ASR, and depending on the circumstances, she too risks developing PTSD.

Esther was a robust, active woman in her seventies whose husband died suddenly when he collapsed in the living room of his home. As her family physician, I was concerned when a year later she still had not recovered her zest for life. One day I asked her to describe the circumstances of his death, slowly and carefully. Her story took a surprising twist when she recalled the words of the paramedic as he entered the room. She was sitting on the floor holding up her husband and he said, 'Oh, no! You should never do that, he must lay flat.'

Now she began sobbing and cried, 'I killed him, didn't I?'

'No, you didn't,' I responded, as I offered her my perspective that she had been a loving spouse and a superlative caregiver who had only been doing her job of supporting her husband when he needed her.

Catastrophic illness or accident

Scattered reports in the literature point to serious illness as a cause of ASR and PTSD. Myocardial infarction,[14] spontaneous abortion,[15] traumatic birth,[16] HIV,[17] diagnosis of cancer,[18] and serious accident[19] have all been reported to do so.

Domestic violence and sexual abuse

The incidence of this is far greater than ever imagined a few decades ago. In the 1980s, Dr Diana Russell created a stir when she interviewed over 900 women and found that one in four had been raped, and one in three sexually abused in childhood.[20]

This form of chronic trauma tends to create helplessness, inaction, limited ability for social engagement, and multiple somatic symptoms in its victims. Often the symptoms are vague, and connection to the underlying trauma long lost.

Unless medical students (and physicians) are specifically trained, they tend to have limited awareness and understanding of domestic violence.[21]

The resident was perplexed. 'This young woman has had a full workup for vague abdominal pain; nothing shows up, yet here she is again. What do I do now?'

I went to speak with her. She didn't seem upset and even bantered with us. She seemed remarkably relaxed, even when I asked her about her significant relationships.

'Well, my boyfriend slaps me around now and then, but only when he's drunk,' she reassured us.

When I suggested that this might possibly have something to do with her pain, she agreed to explore this possibility further. I asked the resident to fetch a chair. We would try the empty chair technique.

'I'd like you to imagine that your boyfriend is in this chair and you need to talk to him about his hitting you. Before we begin, where should I place it?'

She turned pale, and said, 'Not in this room. I want him outside.' I placed the chair just outside the door. She was OK with that, though she wanted the door partially shut.

'Now tell him he is never to hit you again,' I instructed her.

She could barely speak. When she found her voice, it was no more than a whisper. I reassured her it was safe to speak up and with further encouragement she ended up screaming at him, 'You bastard, you ****, you will never do that again. Never again, you hear!'

The resident was wide-eyed and stood with his jaw dropped in total disbelief. The patient too seemed surprised at the vehemence of her reaction. She then agreed to be evaluated by a local organization that assists battered women.

Life-threatening illness prone to recurrence or complications

Most traumas create flashbacks to the events around the incident. With ongoing life-threatening illnesses, such as cancer, that are prone to recurrences and complications, there may be flashbacks and nightmares related to *future* traumas. As one mother of a teenage patient with Hodgkin's lymphoma reported:

It's like a train on a circular track. You are knocked down, and then as you get up, you get knocked down again. You live in terror of every result, every symptom. The future is so frightening.

Who is susceptible

Not everyone exposed to a major trauma develops a traumatic stress disorder. Some are at greater risk than others. Women are more likely to get a stress disorder, particularly when the trauma is rape, as are those who respond to trauma with dissociation rather than action. Individuals who were previously traumatized are susceptible to being retraumatized.

Studies have shown that a significant number of young people enter medical school already traumatized.

- In a confidential survey of 472 medical students done by the Medical College of Wisconsin:
  - 53% reported experiencing severe violence
  - 30%, severe child physical abuse
  - 6%, severe child sexual abuse by family member
  - 13%, child sexual abuse by non-family member
  - 22%, severe partner violence
  - 7%, adult sexual assault.[22]
- An anonymous 70-item questionnaire was sent to 390 first-year medical students at three New England medical schools: 370 students responded, and of these 38% reported personal histories of abuse.[23]

- An anonymous survey involved 406 medical students and 917 full-time faculty: 12.6% reported physical and/or sexual abuse from a partner as adults; 15.0% reported the abuse as a child; 23.9% reported abuse during their lifetime.[24]

When these young people enter medical school they encounter not healing but an environment that has been described as, 'a neglectful and abusive family system', one that is, 'often characterized by their unrealistic expectations, denial, indirect communication patterns, rigidity, and isolation.'[25]

Medical training is intense, chronically stressful, and frequently abusive. With sleep deprivation, education through shame, neglect of personal needs, it bears more than a little resemblance to a marine boot camp except that it lasts years rather than months.

When traumas do occur, physicians are reluctant to seek help. The prevailing environment makes it unsafe to share information. It may affect licensing, credentialing, and be discoverable in pending litigation. At the very least, colleagues are likely to be dismissive.

Response to patients with trauma may be inappropriate, e.g., previously traumatized students become stressed when they encounter violence in others and '... may react by withdrawal, denial, or "intrusive" actions, such as rescue attempts or boundary violations.'[26]

As for patients, we have already seen that there is a high incidence of domestic abuse and sexual abuse in the general public. Traumas sufficient to trigger stress disorders are also surprisingly prevalent. The incidence of exposure to serious traumatic events for adults in USA has been reported as 60.7% in men and 51.2% for women, and 92.2% for men and 87.1% for women in another study.[27] Those subsets of people who are permanently affected are now primed to be retraumatized in subsequent situations.

Additional factors that affect physicians include excessive rigidity and perfectionism, high expectations, abusive litigation system, over-identification with profession.

Practice points

Reject the culture of denial

If you are to develop genuine empathy, then you will need to sensitize yourself to the very real trauma that exists in your environment, whether in yourself, your colleagues, or your patients. The trauma might seem relatively minor (to you, but perhaps not to the person involved) or it might be catastrophic, such as a life-threatening illness, accident, act of violence, or natural disaster, or in the case of a physician, a medical mistake or act of litigation. The trauma may be recent or date back many decades.

Practice prevention

It has been shown that individuals who are most resistant to stress are those who are sociable, have a thoughtful and active coping style, and a strong sense of their ability to control their destiny. You have invested time and money in your education, now invest in yourself. Ask the following questions.

- Am I a loner?
- Do I assign control of my destiny to others?
- Am I a perfectionist?
- Do I tend to beat up on myself when I miss the mark?
- Is my primary identity that of physician?
- Do I lack a community of support?
- Do I lack stress reduction practices?
- Do I suffer from burnout?
- Do I have a history of serious trauma?

If your answer to several of these is yes, then you are probably at greater risk of developing stress disorders. Begin the process of attending to your personal needs and well-being now.[1]

Be prepared

Sooner or later you will have to deal with catastrophic trauma either to yourself or a patient or both. For example, if you are an obstetrician you will inevitably have a stillbirth or death of a newborn. Have a support team that you can draw upon to provide assistance to the mother and her spouse. This might include an appropriate clergyperson or chaplain, social worker, psychologist specializing in trauma, representative of a relevant support group.

Anticipate that trauma victims will react either with stunned silence or highly emotionally. Provide a safe private environment for expression of grief, whatever it is. Remember that cultural factors influence how grief is expressed, and avoid judging the emotions expressed by anyone having a grief reaction. Do not attempt to stifle or hush it.

Treat appropriately

Regardless of type of trauma, principles of treatment are always the same.

- *Establish safety.* Focus on nurturing a safe accepting environment for your patients so that they know that they can express themselves freely, in private and that their story will not denied or judged. Create a calm soothing ambience in your office. Rather than use a highly impersonal *patient registration form* or *interval history form* purchased from a catalog, develop your own. Use language that embraces rather than distances and effectively communicate your practice philosophy.
- *Reconstruct the trauma story.* Should the traumatic event have been a catastrophic incident, ask for the telling of it to be done slowly, as if playing a movie frame by frame. Ask for details of sights, sounds, smells, bodily sensations such as heart rate, as well as feelings experienced at the time. The aim of the story telling is not catharsis; rather it is for the purpose of integration.
- *Restore the connection between survivor and community.* Since trauma is inherently isolating, your connection plays a vital role in rebuilding trust, connection, and meaning. While you cannot necessarily alter the events that have occurred, your willingness to listen and be present can be truly healing, particularly when combined with unexpected acts of kindness on your part.

Following an acute severe trauma, for example a patient whose spouse has suddenly died, advise the following, taking care to do it in writing, or in the presence of a relative or friend.

- You may not be able to think clearly for a while and this is a normal response to an abnormal event. In most cases, symptoms settle down. Label the condition; this is reassuring.
- If you feel stunned, bewildered, and overwhelmed, give yourself time to become grounded. Above all, be gentle with yourself.
- Avoid doing complex tasks or making important decisions during this time.
- Take care of your physical health. This is not a time to perpetuate old habits of sleep deprivation, lack of exercise, working long hours, and indulging in irregular eating habits.
- Try to maintain a familiar, if moderated, schedule. If necessary, take time off from work.
- Do not isolate yourself. Share your experience with those you can trust. If necessary, consult an individual who is trained to listen therapeutically even though deep psychotherapy does not really have a place in the treatment of ASD.
- Limit your use of substances (such as sedatives, hypnotics, alcohol) and limit activities (e.g. burying yourself in work, exercise) aimed at numbing your emotions.

- Conserve your energy. You have only limited control over events. You can, however, apply your energy to improving your well-being.
- If you develop symptoms of depression, do not hesitate to seek professional help and certainly do not attempt to self-medicate.
- Your loved ones are affected by your traumas. They must attend to their own self-care as well.
- Grieving and mourning your losses is healthy and appropriate. Losses unfold slowly, and you may be caught off guard by losses and grief that overcome you when you think you have recovered.

Some further thoughts regarding working with trauma victims:

- Notice the fixed smile, overly quick 'things are fine' response. This may be a mask, behind which is pent-up grief.
- Maintain a high index of suspicion for chronic trauma. Patients with vague complaints, undiagnosed abdominal pain, chronic somatic symptoms, may be suffering from chronic traumatic stress. Very often ASR and PTSD are underdiagnosed and undertreated.[2]
- Traumatized patients tend to be hypervigilant and hypersensitive to non-verbal communication. Be as conscious of your presence, speech, tone of voice, and body language as you are of your speech.
- Even though trauma with its suffering is a stimulus to personal growth, you can remind yourself of this, but never say it to someone in the midst of his or her trauma.
- Never ever say, 'I understand how you feel.' You don't and this expression is highly alienating.
- Standard medical care tends to disempower. With trauma particularly, your role is to empower and to offer as much control to the patient as possible.
- Take care of yourself when working with a traumatized population. Cultivate your own supports so that you do not become secondarily traumatized.

References

1   Bub B (2005) The nightmare of litigation: a survivor's true story. *OBG Management*. **17**: 21–7.

2   Guay S, Mainguy N, Marchand A (2002) Disorders related to traumatic events. Screening and treatment. *Can Fam Physician*. **48**: 512–17.

3   Morrison J (2005) DSM-IV made easy. The clinician's guide to diagnosis. http://mysite.verizon.net/res7oqx1/ (accessed 27 June 2005).

4   American Psychiatric Association (1987) *Diagnostic and Statistical Manual of Psychiatric Disorders* (DSM-111) (3e). American Psychiatric Association, Washington, DC.

5   Frayne S, Seaver M, Loveland S *et al.* (2004) Burden of medical illness in women with depression and postraumatic stress disorder. *Arch Intern Med.* **164**: 1306–12.

6   Herman J (1997) *Trauma and Recovery.* Rivers Oram Press, London.

7   Classen C (1999) Acute stress disorder as a predictor of posttraumatic stress symptoms. *Dir Psychiatry.* **19**: 401–16.

8   Physician insurance litigation stress support services. www.phyins.com/pi/claims/stress.html (accessed 27 June 2005).

9   Kennedy J (2002) Physicians' feelings about themselves and their patients. *JAMA.* **287**: 1113.

10 Hendin H, Lipschitz A, Maltsberger J *et al.* (2000) Therapists' reactions to patients' suicides. *Am J Psychiatry.* **157**: 2022–7.

11 Wu AW, McPhee SJ, Christensen JF (1997) Mistakes in medical practice. In: MD Feldman, JF Christensen (eds) *Behavioural Medicine in Primary Care: a practical guide*, pp. 299–306. Appleton and Lange, Stanford Conn.

12 Brennan TA, Leape LL, Laird NM *et al.* (1991) Incidence of adverse events and negligence in hospitalized patients. Results of the Harvard Medical Practice Study 1. *N Engl J Med.* **324**: 370–6.

13 Breslau N, Kessler RC, Chilcoat HD *et al.* (1998) Trauma and posttraumatic stress disorder in the community: the 1996 Detroit Area Survey of Trauma. *Arch Gen Psychiatry.* **55**: 626–32.

14 Thompson RN (1999) Prediction of trauma responses following myocardial infarction (posttraumatic stress disorder). *Dissertation Abstracts International, Section B, The Sciences and Engineering.* **60**: 2965.

15 Bowles SV, James LC, Solursh DS (2000) Acute and post traumatic stress disorder after spontaneous abortion. *Am Fam Physician.* **61**: 1689–96.

16 Reynolds JL (1997) Post-traumatic stress disorder after childbirth: the phenomenon of traumatic birth. *Can Med Assoc J.* **156**: 831–5.

17 Kelly B, Raphael B, Judd F *et al.* (1998) Posttraumatic stress disorder in response to HIV infection. *Gen Hosp Psychiatry.* **20**: 345–52.

18 McGarvey EL, Canterbury RJ, Cohen RB (1998) Evidence of acute stress disorder after diagnosis of cancer. *South Med J.* **91**: 864–66.

19 Carstensen O, Rasmussen K, Hansen ON *et al.* (1999) Development of posttraumatic stress following severe work-related accidents. *Ugeskr laeger.* **161**: 1249–53.

20 Russell DEH (1984) *Sexual Exploitation: Rape, Child Sexual Abuse, and Sexual Harrassment.* Sage, Beverly Hills, CA.

21 Ernst AA, Houry D, Nick TG (1998) Domestic violence awareness and prevalence in a first-year medical school class. *Acad Emerg Med.* **5**: 64–8.

22 Ambuel B, Butler D, Hamberger LK *et al.* (2003) Female and male students' exposure to violence: impact on well being and perceived capacity to help battered women. *J Comp Fam Stud.* **34**: 113–35.

23 Cullinane PM, Alpert EJ, Freund KM (1997) First-year medical students' knowledge of, attitudes toward, and personal histories of family violence. *Acad Med.* **72**: 315.

24 deLahunta E, Tulsky A (1996) Personal exposure of faculty and medical students to family violence. *JAMA.* **275**: 1903–6.

25 *Family Medicine* (1989) Medical education: a neglectful and abusive family system. November–December.

26 Henricks-Matthews MK (1997) Ensuring students' well-being as they learn to support victims of violence. *Acad Med.* **72**: 46–7.

27 *Primary Psychiatry* (2001) Posttraumatic stress disorder. October.

12

What to listen for: shame

And the two of them were naked, the man and the woman,
and they were not embarrassed.

Genesis 3:1

Then the two ate fruit from the tree of knowledge.
'And the eyes of the two of them were opened, and they knew
   that they were naked.'

Genesis 3:7

We all have those moments when we wake up from our slumber in the Garden of Eden and become self-conscious. Whether it is our bodies, thoughts, values, or behavior, we become aware of aspects of ourselves that make us feel vulnerable and exposed. This is shame and it is the price we pay for having awareness.

Shame is a negative feeling relating to ourselves, *who and how we are*. Guilt is closely related, but refers to a negative feeling about our impact on our environment, i.e., about *what we do to others rather than what we are.*

As infants we are unaware of *self* (like Adam and Eve our 'nakedness' does not bother us), but then, as we mature, we learn to differentiate between *what is me* and *what is not me*. We encounter values in our environment (don't eat from the tree of knowledge) and we internalize them, often unconsciously. Should we act in a way that runs counter to these values, then we experience guilt at having behaved badly, but also some shame at our imperfection and having been found wanting.

When we enter a new environment, either we encounter acceptance, connection, and support, or we experience rejection. The awareness of this rejection may be experienced as shame. Feelings of shame cause us to pause, self-reflect, and alter our behavior. This is *healthy shame*: it is an innately human, normal, self-protective response that grounds us to our values and modulates our behavior accordingly. Shame is part of a feedback loop that regulates our connection with the world and protects our boundaries and our dignity.

There is a spectrum to the experience of shame. It varies from shyness — the sensation of a mild everyday chagrin; to embarrassment with blushing, aversion of one's eyes, and withdrawal; to feelings of humiliation, anger, and panic, with an urge to flee and disappear. This range of response depends on one's relationship to shame. Shame is so ubiquitous in human experience that many labels are given to all its variants. In addition to *shyness, embarrassment, humiliation, chagrin* we encounter words such as *feeling ridiculous, sheepishness, discomfort, disconcertedness, abasement, disgrace, ignominy, dishonor, mortification, degradation, self-consciousness*, etc.[1] The absence of shame is pathological and indicates an individual with Antisocial Personality Disorder.[2]

Not all shame is normal and healthy. *Toxic shame* refers to shame that makes one feel seriously defective, unworthy and inferior. Rather than being supportive, the inner voice may be judgmental, critical and harsh.

The evolution of toxic shame

A child runs to her mother, proudly showing her the scribbles she has done in her mother's favorite coffee-table art book. Her mother can react in various ways.

In one scenario, she might smile and say, 'Wow. How clever, and here is a drawing book for you so in future, you have your very own book to make beautiful pictures. You see, mummy's books are only for reading.' In this interaction the child learns about her mother's value system regarding books, and her self-esteem is left intact. She develops a healthy relationship to shame. If years later, as a teenager, she unconsciously doodles on her mother's book then notices what she has done, she might experience guilt for her behavior and some shame at her-*self* for not being aware. This appropriate level of guilt and shame causes her to apologize and become more careful in the future.

In another scenario, her mother might react in horror and scream, 'Bad girl, you ruined my favorite book. I keep telling your father how rotten you kids are.' Here she learns that she is bad and defective as a person. If as a teenager she discovers herself doodling in a book, her internalized shame is triggered and there is no need for her mother to harp on her 'badness' since her own inner critic reminds her of this. When asked about the book, she reacts defensively denying responsibility, and lashes out in anger. No-one suspects that underlying toxic shame is responsible for her behavior. It is embarrassing to *admit I feel shame* so her tendency is to react with other emotions such as anger, rage, or cynicism, thereby masking the shame. Attacks of anger trigger more shame, and shame spirals. She withdraws from the environment that has been so rejecting thinking, 'I don't need them; I can manage on my own.' In this way she echoes society's values that adults should be strong, independent, and autonomous. Any feelings of neediness trigger further shame.

Over the years she develops anticipatory shame, i.e., she is so primed for rejection that she anticipates it and tries to organize her life in a way that prevents her from having to experience shame.

Shame, students, and physicians

Imagine this young woman develops a desire to do healing work and enters medical school. She usually tries to be invisible in one of the back rows of the auditorium, but one day she arrives late and is forced to sit up front during a clinical presentation. To her horror, the professor calls her out to examine a patient in front of her entire class.

'Doctor' – Prof. Smith always refers to medical students as doctor, perhaps to emphasize that they are not one – 'what do you think of this patient's eye?'

All 150 pairs of eyes stare down from the seats in the auditorium glued onto this unfortunate medical student unlucky enough to have been plucked from the front row.

'The pupil is … ah … fixed and dilated. It doesn't react to light or accommodation. I think he is blind in this eye sir, I'm not sure why.'

'Brilliant deduction, doctor you have diagnosed your first prosthetic eye.'

Everyone laughs as she turns scarlet.

I was a member of that class 36 years ago, and I remember it as if it were yesterday. This was just one of many lessons that were indelibly branded into our memories. Shame, in those days, was used as powerful teaching tool.

Most physicians experience shame during their training as medical students and during their years in practice. As we have seen, medical students are often shamed by their perceived inadequacies. There are many levels of hierarchy in hospitals and here lowly residents are ranked just above students. Residents are often overworked, sleep-deprived and, being in training, often make errors. They cannot ask for assistance since this implies weakness and is itself shameful. The result of errors is abuse and perhaps litigation. Physicians in practice make mistakes and then may feel toxic shame. As litigation defendants, they are attacked by patients, their families, and opposing attorneys, and occasionally even by their own insurers.

It is the nature of shame that the incidents that most stand out in our memories are those that are traumatic or feel shameful.

Anna is an internist. One day during her residency, she was particularly anxious to get home. Her last patient of the day was a priest. He was talking to her while she was drawing his blood. She interrupted him to remove the tourniquet and apply a Band-aid. As she stood up to leave he asked her, 'Doctor, aren't you going to let me finish my story?' She felt intense shame. How could she not listen to him? This incident occurred in 1958 and was still painful to the teller, now retired, in 2004.

Jerome is a nephrologist. He tends to perfectionism – his immaculate appearance of gold-rimmed glasses, cuff links, highly polished shoes, and sharply pressed trousers attests to that. One day a resident saw him altering his previous day's note in the patient's hospital chart. He was reported and reprimanded. 'The shame of it, the shame of it,' he wept as he shared this incident with me.

I have my own experiences that are vividly emblazoned in my memory. A mother brought her 7-year-old son into the office. He had suddenly lost his vision in both eyes. His pupils reacted just fine, but he seemed totally blind. I was perplexed so rushed him to the emergency room to see an ophthalmologist. While waiting, a nurse came along, older and much wiser than me. She offered the little boy a candy bar and he reached for it enthusiastically. We cancelled the ophthalmologist and called the psychiatrist.

In the practice of medicine, there are many potential missteps that can lead to shame when a physician feels that he failed.[3] James Kennedy MD, in a letter to *JAMA*, even suggested that he believes toxic shame is responsible for PTSD in most physicians.[4]

There are many ramification of shame in physicians. For example, one way of avoiding shame is to do it pre-emptively to others, in effect *shame or be shamed*. Who would suspect that a physician who is obnoxious, condescending, and insensitive to patients, ancillary staff, and employees may himself be suffering from toxic shame? This may explain at least some bizarrely inappropriate comments made by physicians.

Suicide is another issue. Even though other causes of death tend to be lower in physicians, the incidence of suicide has climbed to a level significantly higher than in non-physicians. In a study of suicide notes in general, three-quarters contained the theme of apology/shame.[5] There has not been a study of suicide notes of physicians, but it is tempting to think that isolation, trauma, and shame may have a role to play in a large percentage of cases. This is a serious public health issue, yet no definitive study has been done on suicide incidence in physicians in the USA in the past 20 years.[6]

Perhaps this is a case of the profession's shame?

Shame and patients

At least physicians do not have to expose their vulnerabilities. Patients do have to expose theirs. Secrets, whether physical or emotional, are revealed. Bodily functions normally private, are subject to interrogation and exposed. Disfigurements normally disguised are placed under the spotlight. All of this may induce shame. The lack of sensitivity by even well-intentioned physicians can be appalling.

> Jenny had had an emergency caesarian section which left her with a badly scarred abdomen. She was very self-conscious of this. Another gynecologist saw her later. Her retort was, 'This looks awful. You should sue the guy. Your belly looks like a railroad track!'

Some people have a lifetime of shame related to a birth defect or deformities. It takes courage to face the world when one is exquisitely sensitive about one's appearance.

> One couple found happiness. Each had a harelip but they found acceptance in each other. They had a baby – sadly, it too was born with a harelip. The obstetrician could not deal with this. He thrust the baby into the arms of the nurse and stormed off exclaiming, 'This baby is cursed!' The mother, now in her eighties, still remembers how what was to have been the happiest day of her life was transformed into an indelible trauma.

Patients are fearful, dependent, and sometimes helpless. As a society we value independence and autonomy. The very nature of being a patient is to be dependent and needy. When a patient has pre-existing toxic shame, the effects of illness may be magnified.

Richard had a herniated disk with incapacitating sciatica. He was a truck driver, 45 years old and had never previously missed a day's work due to illness in his life. Placed on absolute bed rest, he chain smoked, snacked, gained weight and was absolutely miserable.

'Why are you so upset?' I asked.

'You don't understand doc. I have been working since I was 14 years old. Now I feel like worthless trash. I am no use to my family or anybody.'

'What do you mean, worthless trash?' I asked, shocked at the vehemence of his response.

'My father used to put a belt to me. He taught me right. A man has to work and support his family and there is no place in this world for idleness.'

Richard required sedation, the shame was so great.

Frequently patients see their physicians for emotional or stress-related reasons often involving shameful situations, e.g., divorce. Those experiencing shame, e.g., a fired employee or a divorcee, may remain loners, but most shift to other environments hoping to find support and validation rather than rejection and denigration.

Gordon Wheeler writes that the search for a new environment involves '... new outreach and support coming from some significant person or group in the field (such as the listening of a friend, the extraordinary holding we extend to people in states of sudden loss, or the relational process of psychotherapy).'[7]

Frequently this search for support involves the healthcare professional. We all have people in our lives whom we consider safe – they are our support team. *My lawyer, my accountant, my minister or rabbi, my doctor – I can tell them what bothers me. I may be feeling rejected by everyone else but I can at least count on their empathetic support. If I am feeling very sensitive, then just a hint of criticism from them is particularly distressing to me.*

The important point to note is that while patients seek objectivity and skill from their physicians, there is always a hidden agenda involving the need to be accepted and supported – a hidden agenda that is not satisfied by objective professionalism.

Practice points

- You cannot know the HIV status of a patient by external appearance alone. Similarly, you cannot know the shame predisposition of an individual by appearance alone. As with HIV, assume that every person is easily shamed until proven otherwise.
- A basic requirement for healing is that you do not traumatize by inadvertently adding to shame where it already exists.
- Create an environment of safety and support where everyone is treated with dignity and respect. When you need to review errors or other problems with employees or colleagues, do it privately and at professional meetings. Be careful to separate behavior from self.
- A major part of the medical education process involves giving feedback to students and residents. Giving honest and clear feedback without stimulating shame in the process is a major challenge for you if you are a teacher or employer. Some shame is almost inevitable, but the aware teacher will never do it deliberately, and will also take care to simultaneously provide support.
- Your acceptance and non-judgmental behavior can be very healing. Notice if you feel distaste or disgust, and appreciate that your patient has probably received such a response from others.
- Train your employees. Even the most seemingly innocent remark 'hmmmm, we gained a little weight didn't we' embarrasses someone who is highly self-conscious about her weight.
- Medicine utilizes language that is unintentionally shaming: mitral incompetence, respiratory failure, renal impairment, decompensated liver disease, incompetent cervix, ovarian failure, vitamin deficiency, weak bladder, etc. Use terminology consciously.
- Humor is invaluable when working with people. Be very careful never to use humor at a patient's expense even if you think it is really, really funny.
- Be particularly sensitive of someone with a long-standing disability, deformity, or disfigurement. You may be objective, but a patient cannot possibly be.
- When you encounter a patient with such a condition, appreciate that you cannot eliminate their shame. What you can do is to provide safety, build trust, and relationship, and eventually your patient may open up to you and express shame that until now has been kept from the world. This presents a special opportunity for healing.
- If you have experienced toxic shame, notice whether you are signaling to others your need for their approval and acceptance. This may make you vulnerable to others taking unfair advantage of you.

References

1   Lee R (1994) Couples shame: The unaddressed issue. In: G Wheeler and S Backman (eds) *On Intimate Ground: a Gestalt approach to working with couples.* Jossey-Bass, San Francisco.

2   *Primary Psychiatry* (2001) Antisocial Personality Disorder: the forgotten patients of psychiatry, pp. 30–54. January.

3   Cunningham W, Wilson H (2003) Shame, guilt and the medical practitioner. *N Z Med J.* **116**: U629.

4   Kennedy J (2002) Physicians' feelings about themselves and their patients. *JAMA.* **287**: 1113–14.

5   Foster T (2003) Suicide note themes and suicide prevention. *Int J Psychiatry Med.* **33**: 323–31.

6   Center C, Davis M, Detre T *et al.* (2003) Confronting depression and suicide in physicians: a consensus statement. *JAMA.* **289**: 3161–6.

7   Wheeler G (1997) Self and shame: a Gestalt approach. *Gestalt Review.* **1**: 221–44.

13

What to listen for: *suffering*

Love is a toil and life is a trouble
Riches will fade and beauty will flee
Pleasures they dwindle and prices they double
And nothing is as I would wish it to be.
                    Housewife's lament, c. 19th century[1]

'If only I hadn't fallen down the steps and fractured my ankle.'
'If only I had my health and youth back again.'
'If only Medicare didn't keep changing the rules.'
'If only I could practice medicine the way I did in the old days.'

Suffering is the one narrative theme that permeates the entire healthcare system and, as such, spares few patients and professionals. Trauma (and illness is a trauma) results in suffering and people who suffer cry, mourn, wail, complain, moan, i.e., they lament. Usually the lament is vocal and obvious; not infrequently, however, it is non-verbal with a sigh, a slump of the shoulders, a shrug, or a tear. A lament may be hidden in a cynical comment, a joke, an angry outburst, or it may be borne in silence. The lament may also manifest as chronic fatigue or multiple functional somatic symptoms. In other words, a lament is transmitted in many guises. No matter how it manifests, however, the lament is always an expression of suffering.

Hidden though it may be, suffering is a universal human condition and its symptom, the lament, can almost always be recognized if the listener knows what to listen for. Identifying the lament is essential if the listener is to consistently demonstrate empathy and understanding.

This was dramatically demonstrated to me on a recent journey I took to Canada, ironically to present a workshop based on this very topic. It began with a visit to the photocopy store.

The assistant

Oh dear, I don't want to spend the whole day waiting to copy some handouts for this workshop. I noticed my own lament seeping out as I saw the store overflowing with disgruntled customers waiting for service. Finally, I caught the eye of one of the two overwhelmed employees.

Setting aside my own frustration, I commented, 'You seem to be very busy today.'

'Oh, you should see us on weekends,' she replied.

'Why, does it get worse than this?' I asked rhetorically, my lament 'light bulb' having gone off.

'Ha! This is nothing! We're often even more short-staffed then when employees don't show up,' she replied.

'It must be very challenging for you,' I suggested empathetically.

She responded with a vigorous nod.

From then on, her lament having been heard and validated, I had her full attention. She led me to a working copier and then stopped by every few minutes to check that things were OK, each time adding to her story: 'You know they should have a mechanic on duty, these machines keep breaking down ... and why can't they have someone on call in event an employee doesn't show up for work ... and why ...'

The bed and breakfast hostess

Since the workshop on laments was to be given in Vancouver, Canada, en route we stayed over at a quaint bed and breakfast in a small town in the Canadian Rockies.

The following morning at breakfast, our hostess, neatly dressed in a white chef's outfit, proudly presented us with an Irish breakfast. And then, having discovered I was a physician, hovered and hovered, and hovered, endlessly rambling on about her arthritis and chronic fatigue syndrome, not to mention the inadequacies of her physicians, all the while our eggs growing cold. Suddenly, I had an *Aha!*

'How do you manage to run a bed and breakfast in your condition, with all these beds, stairs, meals and so forth? It must be very difficult with your knees being so painful,' I commented empathetically.

An expression of long-suffering resignation took over. 'It's hard, really hard,' she sighed. 'Thank you for listening, I'll run along now, mustn't keep you from your breakfast or it will get cold.'

Off she toddled, her face beaming, her lament having been heard and validated.

The psychiatrist
After a few days of sightseeing, we arrived in Vancouver. Some friends, happy to see us, organized a small dinner party the night before the conference. Seated opposite me was a psychiatrist.
'Why are you here in Vancouver?' she asked.
'To teach communication skills to physicians' I replied.
'Good luck!' she snapped. 'They constantly refer patients to me without even a brief note of introduction. Communication skills, ha! I've tried everything, it doesn't help!'
'It must be very hard for you,' I replied, 'how do you cope?'

Each of these three individuals encountered on my journey to the workshop expressed a lament. Each had a complaint that included elements of hopelessness, helplessness and disempowerment. Each unconsciously needing to have the lament heard, appreciated for what it was, and validated.

A lament can even more subtle:

The fellow
Returning from presenting at a conference, I found myself sharing a cab to the railway station with a young medical fellow. As we pulled up to the station, she commented, 'I hope the train is on time. Amtrak is often late.'

She sighed and repeated, 'Yes, they're erratic'.

While we waited for the train, which incidentally arrived on time, she asked what I taught.
'Listening skills to physicians — for example, how to recognize a lament,' I responded.
'What is a lament?' she asked.
'You just did it, a few minutes ago,' I replied.
She looked at me quizzically.
'Remember your comment about Amtrak, that was a lament. You sighed as you said it, and you repeated yourself. You know when a word or a phrase is repeated in the Bible, it's always significant. Same in real life. Neither of us wants the train to be late, but for you it has a special significance.'

We seated ourselves across the aisle from one another. She chatted easily about her job. How fortunate she was to have it. It required some travel, but was otherwise a 'plum'. There were many perks, such as her recent 8 weeks maternity leave instead of the usual six. 'Yes,' she continued, 'my friends envy me having a job I actually enjoy, something unusual in this day and age.'

'How old is your baby?' I asked.

'She's eight months old, the joy of my life. My husband's babysitting. She will be asleep by the time I get home, I guess,' she replied with a sigh, her smile now less pronounced.

'Is it hard for you to be away from them?' I asked.

'It is,' she said, her voice now soft. 'It's been tough. Still, it's too good a job to give up.' Her eyes were misty.

Leaning forward across the aisle toward her, in an invisible 'bubble' of rapport, I suggested that it had to be wrenching making the choice between work and baby. Regardless how great the job, her losses were big. She nodded, silent now.

After a while I asked, 'What will you do with the next one?'

'No way will I return to work!' her voice now assertive and strong. She then paused for a moment, 'So, I was lamenting, ha? I had no idea.'

When the time came for me to disembark, she flashed a broad goodbye smile. She was sitting straighter. Lightness had come over her.

If the response to suffering is the lament, then surely patients have much to lament about as they experience trauma and losses from their illnesses, aggravated by the additional layers of trauma and suffering inflicted by the often impersonal, expensive, and complex healthcare system. It is not surprising therefore that the term *patient* is derived from the Latin word *patiens* meaning 'to suffer'.

When a patient has a complaint, the usual response of a physician is to either reassure or attempt to treat the underlying condition. The effective response for a lament however, is totally counterintuitive and involves neither reassurance nor problem solving. This makes the recognition of a lament particularly important.

Some historical background to laments

Classically laments are found in the Biblical book of Lamentations which mourns the fall of the first temple in 587 BCE and the exile of the Jewish people to Babylon, and in the book of Job, the ultimate sufferer. These books are suffused with themes of loneliness, abandonment, absence of meaning, suffering, sin, and guilt. The book of Psalms, too, contains examples of laments. Some biblical examples are:

- *'I am disgusted with life; I will give reign to my complaint, speak in the bitterness of my soul.'* (Job 10:1)
- *'Bitterly she weeps at night, tears upon her cheek. With not one to console her ...'* (Lamentations 1:2)
- *I call God to mind, I moan, I complain, my spirit fails.* (Psalm 77:4).

Physicians too have a long history of laments, mostly ones that center on demands of patients or despair over harsh working conditions. For example, Maimonides in the 13th century wrote in a letter to a friend:

> *My duties to the Sultan are very heavy. I am obliged to visit him every day, early in the morning, and when he or any of his children or concubines are indisposed, I cannot leave Cairo but must stay during most of the day ... When night falls, I am so exhausted I can hardly speak.*[2]

Over the years, patients have viewed physicians as both a blessing and a curse. The price of cure is often additional suffering imposed on patients by expensive, uncomfortable, and sometimes painful treatments. It is not surprising, therefore, that physicians have always been the butt of patient laments:

> *When you are in need of a physician, you esteem him like a god; when he has brought you out of danger, consider him a kin; when you have been cured he becomes human like yourself; when he sends his bill you think of him as a devil.* (Jedaiah Berdesi, 14th century.)[3]

> *The angel of death was in need of help so he appointed doctors as his deputies.* (Reb Nachman of Breslov, 18th century.)[4]

Or as Chekhov famously put it:

> *Doctors are just the same as lawyers; the only difference is that lawyers merely rob you, whereas doctors rob and kill you too.*

The situation today

Nowadays the public can be heard to complain about their medical care in coffee shops, restaurants, in public transport, and certainly anywhere that elderly people congregate – or to me, when they hear the title of my book.

Physicians in turn lament their many losses in the healthcare revolution,[5,6] and the pressures of managed care, over-regulation, and the treadmill of practice that provide insufficient time to spend with patients. This incessant complaining has been described by JN Brouilette, MD, as the *Physician Moaning Syndrome*.[7] He states that this syndrome can be found in its most severe form wherever physicians congregate, e.g., doctors' lounges. There, he writes, 'They complain of chronic fatigue, depression, and loss of self-esteem.'

What specifically is a lament?

Simply stated, a lament is an expression of suffering, a crying out of pain — physical, emotional, and spiritual. The Hebrew title for the book of Lamentations is *Eikhah*, meaning 'How?' The rough guttural G sound of this word embodies the harshness of the pain. The lament contains some elements of hopelessness, helplessness, disempowerment, absence of choice, pessimism, grief, weariness, lack of meaning, and isolation from others, from God, and from self. It might also include anger, fear, shame, anguish, self-blame, guilt, or cynicism.

Paradoxically, it also includes hope, since in lamenting, the individual is reaching out from a place of isolation, with the unconscious hope that the cry will be heard. The ultimate state of despair and loss of faith is found in a person who *cannot* lament. Hence, behind the incorrigible optimist may be someone who does not experience the luxury to express mourning or the never-complaining individual who unexpectedly commits suicide.

The lament is really more than an expression, rather is part of the experience and new reality. 'The delicate dance between expression and experience continues interdependently, each leading, each following, each birthing the other.'[8] Sometimes the lament seems to take over the very identity of the individual with a telling and retelling of the trauma for years after the event. In this case, there is little that the listener can say or do that impacts the lamenter since it is so ingrained in the personality.

The lament may be written, drawn, spoken, sung, wailed, cried, mimed, danced, shrugged, laughed, or borne in silence. It may also be expressed as physical symptoms. At least 33% of somatic symptoms are medically unexplained, and these symptoms are chronic or recurrent in 20% to 25% of patients. There is a strong coexistence of anxiety and depression in these patients.[9] It is conceivable that many suffering from chronic multiple functional somatic symptoms are in fact lamenting.

A lament takes one of two forms, acute or chronic:

The acute lament

The acute lament is a normal, healthy, integral part of the healing process. In the face of sudden severe losses, crying, bemoaning, and wailing serve to generate the energy that frees the individual from the numbness created by the shock of trauma, and allows the traumatized individual to adjust and realign to the new reality.

Alternatively, with overwhelming trauma, the response may be stunned, numbed, silence, not necessarily lament but rather the Acute Stress Reaction (ASR).

The chronic lament

In the usual course of events, trauma leads to a sequence of events that I call the *Healing Sequence.*

The healing sequence

Trauma → *Losses* → *Suffering* → *Lamenting* → *Listening* → *Healing*

For example, an elderly lady has a stroke. This illness is a *trauma*. It results in *losses* of strength, function, autonomy, mobility, independence, self-esteem, etc. These losses have to be endured and the consequence is *suffering*. When her doctor visits her in the nursing home she is despondent and has a multitude of complaints. These are her *laments*. He is astute, so he *listens* and focuses on cultivating their relationship. Eventually, she begins to look forward to his visits even though he does not cure her. Rather than disempowering her with his suggestions, he empowers her by asking her what she needs so that they form a partnership in her care. An element of *healing* has begun.

Etiology of a chronic lament

A lament may become chronic when grief following an acute trauma is interrupted, disowned, or disenfranchised, and there is no opportunity for complete mourning. It may also occur when the onset of trauma is gradual or trauma is unrelenting. In all cases, the *Healing Sequence* is interrupted.

The traumas leading to the chronic lament experienced in medical practice may be dramatic and obvious; mostly they are not. The mother of a sick child, the spouse of an Alzheimer patient, the patient with an arthritic knee, the doctor fighting managed care, the underappreciated receptionist, the overworked nurse — all experience traumas and losses, and tend to lament them chronically.

Being denied the transformative power that comes from openly expressing grief, energy needing to go somewhere seeps out. The poet Rumi described this in the 13th century '... I spill sad energy everywhere. My story gets told in various ways: a romance, a dirty joke, a war, a vacancy.'[10]

Certain groups of individuals are at higher risk for laments – the recently separated or divorced, the unemployed, patients, particularly the elderly. The nursing home patient for example, expressing one complaint after the other, may cause a less astute physician to scramble to treat each physical symptom in turn, not realizing that the patient is lamenting losses of home, friends, family, mobility, independence, etc. Eventually he dreads seeing the patient. The result is that the *physician* feels inadequate, frustrated, and angry, and the *patient* is disgruntled and asks for another physician.

Some specific examples follow.

Some specific examples

Disenfranchised grief

The supervisor
She is successful, well-liked at work, and enjoys a sense of camaraderie with her colleagues. Much to her delight, she is rewarded with a promotion. Later she notices that the atmosphere at work has subtly changed. She is no longer invited by her former co-workers to join them during coffee breaks. Recently she had to discipline one of them and that was very uncomfortable for her. She feels chronically tired and can't understand why, since she has lots to be thankful for. She visits her doctor for some blood tests. When asked about her life she tells him its fine, she has just been promoted. Eventually she sees a therapist and learns that transitions, even good ones, are always accompanied by some losses. When these losses are not anticipated and mourned, they end up becoming burdens.

The medical resident
The head of the residency program receives reports that one of his physicians demonstrates irritability, sarcasm, and a negative attitude towards nurses and patients. He invites the resident for a walk and talk. He asks about young man's life and learns that the resident, a native of India, comes from a very close-knit family. A few months ago he missed his brother's wedding because he could not take time off to return home. He tells himself he should be used to this by now, after all the years of study in medical school. 'This is the price one pays for being a doctor, isn't it?' he remarks.

The internist
His beeper went off. He excused himself to make a phone call, then returned looking flushed. 'Those damn nurses calling to tell me the patient has constipation after I asked not to be disturbed unless it was an emergency. I shouldn't complain though; as a rehabilitation specialist my patients are paraplegic or worse!'

The family doctor
'You think you have problems! Look at me, I work 12 hours a day, reimbursement is down, work isn't fun anymore. You don't hear me complain.'

Interrupted grief

Sometimes losses are just too great and mourning is just too painful, so rather than immerse in inconsolable grief, some choose to live 'lives of quiet desperation' neither experiencing the depths of despair nor peaks of joy. Others find themselves so overwhelmed with issues that mourning is a luxury they cannot afford.

The widow
There are funeral arrangements to organize, insurances, taxes, finances to sort out. Decisions such as where to live need to be made. It's all so rushed, since his death was unexpected. Weeks fly by, now grief hits in waves. When asked how she is, she switches on a tight smile and responds she's fine. Nights are the hardest, so she visits her doctor regularly to renew her prescription for sleeping pills.

Ongoing trauma

The family physician
A typical successful doctor, he works 60 hours plus a week. Two years ago his wife, who was also his office manager, divorced him. The front office has been a shambles since the new manager doesn't seem to be coping. Their two teenage daughters chose to live with him. This has

been a mixed blessing since they are both acting out, with one failing at school and the other involved with a rough crowd and displaying poor judgment in her choice of boyfriends. He feels he is constantly 'putting out fires'. Much of the time he's tired and cranky. One of his few pleasures is being treated to lunch by those pretty pharmaceutical representatives; at least they listen attentively to him as he shares his frustrations.

Mechanism of a chronic lament

The movement of energy with the chronic lament is *circular and non-linear*. Dr Simcha Raphael, psychotherapist, calls this 'stuck movement' (personal communication). Like a tape recording played over and over, the lament leads nowhere.

The lamenter needing to be heard repeats the lament constantly, often unconsciously and in a number of vague ways. It may also be almost totally masked – the patient with a fixed smile, the always joking physician, the cynic, the intellectual, the loner, the disruptive physician (or patient), the workaholic. Consequently, the lament is frequently missed.

The irony is that the chronic lament is mostly counterproductive, alienating rather than drawing others closer. Like a foreign body in a wound, it draws attention to itself and inhibits healing rather than facilitating it. Only when genuine emotion is felt and expressed can the lament begin to shift into constructive action. In other words, when the chronic lamenter experiences sadness or weeps in the course of talking, this is a positive sign.

Typical response to a lament

The acute lament

When my last doctor gave me the news, I burst into tears. He then ran out of the room to fetch a nurse. You know doctors can't stand suffering! (A former patient)

I was devastated by the news. All I could think of was to ask how long I had to live. About two to four years, the doctor responded perfunctorily as if I had just asked him the time. He shuffled some papers and quickly disappeared. (A cancer patient)

The chronic lament

There is an inherent and mostly unaware need to have one's lament heard and validated. This might occur occasionally, but mostly people find listening to another's chronic complaints a frustrating and challenging experience. At best, laments are usually shrugged off. The letter to one medical journal entitled 'Note to doctors: stop whining'[11] is typical. A column in the *New York Times* went further. Not only did the physician author demonstrate a remarkable lack of empathy to a medical resident's lament of being in a 'chronically nervous state,' she went on to preach that he needed to study and acquire empathy for his patients. Her recipe: 'stay awake every third night for 3 years, tired, aching, nauseated, and terrified that despite the very best intentions in the world you are about to make a terrible mistake.'[12]

So much for empathy! This is the same absurd order of teaching as: *I saw a mother slap her baby so I went up to her and slapped her. Now she'll know not to do it again.*

Many physicians, deprived of empathy themselves, tend to lack the capacity to show empathy for patients. Symptomatic of this, the condition of multiple functional symptoms is labeled somewhat disrespectfully by some as 'The fat folder syndrome' or 'The familiar face syndrome'.

The effective healing response to a lament

This is discussed in depth further on. Suffice to point out that rather than offering advice or attempting to resolve the perceived problem (i.e., adding to the disempowerment) the listener attempts to listen, understand, and validate the focus on building rapport and relationship. This is based on trust that healing will emerge *from the relationship itself* rather from resolution of the issues.

The nursing home patient
(D, doctor; P, patient)
D: How are you today Mrs Cohn? *(D inquiring about her as a person, not her knees.)*
P: Not so good doctor. *(She sighs.)* *(D thinks he hears a lament.)*
D: Why, what's happening? *(D now sits down for better eye contact, signals he intends to listen.)*
P: It's my knees. The medicine you gave me isn't working. Just like the others. *(D momentarily feels annoyed, and silently acknowledges his frustration and then parks it.)*

D: So you are having a lot of pain? *(D acknowledges and invites further response.)*

P: Yes, and it's affecting my bowels. Just can't go every day. *(She pauses. D tolerates this.)*
And every 5 minutes I have to pass my water. The water pills don't help matters.

D: Must be very difficult going to the bathroom with your knees being so painful. *(D is validating her experience.)*

P: You cannot imagine.

D: No, I can't. How do you cope? *(D signals his empathy.)*

P: I have to call the nurse to come help me. And you know what they are like. Always so busy.

D: And you used to be so independent. *(D identifies and labels loss of independence.)*

P: I was. I stood in the grocery store from six in the morning to nine at night. Never asked for help.

D: You have had so many losses in the last few years. *(D making the point she's had more losses.)*

P: Yes. I had to sell my home; such a beautiful house. I lived in it for 40 years, raised all my children in it. They made me sell my car. My friends are dead. Better I should be gone.

D: You feel you are better off dead?

P: Yes *(sobbing now)*, don't worry, I'm not going to do anything.

D: *(after a pause)* This must very painful for you, feeling so helpless. *(D has identified another loss.)*

P: It is. It feels terrible being alone and needing help. Nothing to look forward to. None of my old friends are alive and my family doesn't come by so often anymore. *(Isolation, loneliness, other losses are identified.)*

D: I'm sorry. With you feeling so bad, how can I be most helpful to you? *(D making an empowering suggestion.)*

P: I know you can't take all the pain away, perhaps something I can take once in a while if the pain is too severe. And something for my bowels. Thank you doctor.

D: (taking her hand) OK, I will be happy to do that and I'll see you again in 2 weeks. *(D is saying, in effect, I am here for you.)*

Over the next few months she begins to look forward to his visits. They talk about her former life. He shares a little about his. Compassion emerges. He now appreciates her many losses – independence, pride, empowerment, bodily functions, mobility, relationships, meaning, etc. He recognizes her anger, shame, despair, isolation, and helplessness.

He no longer dreads visiting her, so his own sense of well-being improves. He also finds he has to spend less time fielding calls from the nursing home.[13]

Adapted and reproduced with permission from the BMJ Publishing Group.

With skilled listening, one of the most *frustrating* listening challenges in medicine, the lament, can be transformed into one of the most *rewarding*, i.e., from 'our dancing is changed into mourning' (Lamentations 5:15) to 'you turned my lament into dancing' (Psalm 30:12).

Practice points

Learn to identify a lament

You cannot appropriately treat a medical condition until you first diagnose it. Similarly, you cannot appropriately treat suffering until you hear its symptom, the lament.

Anticipate it

Common things occur commonly, therefore expect to hear expressions of suffering from patients (and healthcare professionals). If individuals have suffered losses expect a lament.

Listen for clues

Watch body language; listen for the use of disempowering words such as *but, can't, should, must* and *if only*. Notice if there is a narrative theme of hopelessness, helplessness, pessimism, weariness, loneliness, or negativity. Do you sense that the person seems trapped in his/her situation?

Notice your own response

Ask yourself the following questions.

- Am I finding myself wanting to avoid this person?
- Do I find myself yawning, bored and irritated as I listen?
- Do I feel redundant here, as if this person doesn't see me?
- Am I hearing a tape and my presence is actually irrelevant?
- Was our conversation highjacked by a lament?
- Do I feel stimulated to offer advice, counsel, or fix a problem?

- Do I notice a mismatch between the power of the story and the emotional flatness of the delivery?

Any of the above suggests you are listening to a lament.

Respond effectively

Once the light bulb goes off – *Aha! I hear a lament*, then treatment of the underlying suffering follows a predictable path. Most healthcare professionals respond instinctively to an issue with reassurance, comfort, or treatment. Remind yourself that physical symptoms can be treated and fixed but *spiritual or emotional suffering requires healing*.

The acute lament

- Appreciate that the open expression of grief is a healthy process and that your prime aim is to make space for it and certainly avoid aborting it.
- Following a major trauma, limit the use of tranquilizers and sedatives, and caution about alcohol intake.
- A quiet supportive presence is helpful, meaningful, and healing.
- Silence may be the best *active* response, since space is being created for grief, with you serving as an invaluable witness to the experience. There are different types of silence – icy, cold, warm, intimate, etc. A helpful image of silence here is one in which 'You hold in your heart the person with whom you are sitting, creating a warm silence where he or she knows you are not off somewhere else in your thoughts' (personal communication, Rabbi Goldie Milgram, MSW).
- Attend to 'simple' details, such as having tissues on hand and ensuring privacy.

Though nothing has been fixed, often long after the event, the sensitive role played by the healthcare professional will be recalled with appreciation.

The chronic lament

Once you recognize that you are listening to a lament, you will feel less helpless and disempowered yourself. Now you know that just your listening and validating is helpful. Remember however to avoid directly labeling what you hear as *a lament*. This distances rather than creates relationship.

You pay particular attention to the following.

- Being fully present and demonstrating this with eye contact, body language, and verbal response.
- Regardless of the temptation, not responding with advice, critique, or reassurance.
- Suspending personal judgment. Each person's suffering is unique. What might seem trivial to you, may feel important to your patient.
- Offering therapeutic validation (the intentional use of validation in ways that enhance the recipient's capacity to face life's existential moments).[14] It requires identifying the underlying emotions, and reflecting back in a way that demonstrates understanding of them.
- Demonstrating empathy with phrases such as 'I am sorry to hear this' or 'What a sad time for you.'
- Being very careful not to respond with, 'I understand,' or 'I know what you are going through,' since it is impossible to fully understand the suffering of another.
- Suspending attachment to outcomes.
- Silently acknowledge your own anxiety at not being totally in control of the length, direction, or outcome of the encounter, and reminding oneself that time listening often feels longer than it is in reality.

When your patient feels heard and validated, the lament tends to fade and the focus of your patient's attention may shift from lament to you the listener. You may actually feel visible as person for the first time in this encounter. Even though you have not fixed anything, a shift has occurred. This may be sufficient for most transient situations. Now your interaction may feel alive for the first time.

If there is an ongoing relationship, then opportunity for further healing exists. Taking healing a step further requires a deeper understanding of the nature of suffering.

The word *suffer* is derived from the Latin *sufferre* – *to carry*. To suffer is *to carry* or *to endure*. What is being carried is always an unwanted weight, i.e., a burden, and usually it feels as if this burden is being carried alone. You may recall that the nature of trauma is to cause alienation and isolation. This understanding of suffering – that it implies carrying a burden and involves isolation – provides you with some specific healing opportunities.

Name the suffering

Responding, 'How do you possibly manage to cope?' or 'You have endured so much, what keeps you going?', or words to that effect, raises the lamenter's awareness (perhaps for the very first time) that he or she is suffering. This awareness alone serves to ease suffering. The renowned philosopher and Holocaust survivor Viktor Frankl articulated it well, 'Emotion, which is suffering, ceases to be suffering when we form a clear and precise picture of it.'[15]

Identify losses

Ask yourself, 'What is this person being forced to carry or endure?' This helps identify losses. Reflected back, this helps the lamenter connect to specific losses, and to move into a phase of conscious mourning, a precondition for moving forward.

Relieve isolation

Not only is a burden being carried, it feels as if it is being carried alone. The very nature of suffering is separation and isolation. This can be understood from the perspective of a cancer patient. The moment the diagnosis is revealed, this person now leaves the community of the healthy and faces an unknown future. Having the lament heard and supported means that this burden is no longer being supported alone.

Shift perception

The lament tape may be played so often that it is experienced as the reality of the situation. This becomes a fixed image. When the listener reflects back what is heard, e.g., 'So you *feel* you have only one choice,' this may stimulate awareness that this is a feeling and not necessarily reality. Images may shift. The question, 'What do you think you need right now?' may sharpen the focus from lament to specific need and transform aimless lament into action.

Empower

Powerlessness, helplessness is the lamenter's present reality. It is rarely absolute. Asking 'What supports or strengths do you have?' may help the lamenter connect with forgotten strengths. Asking 'How may I be most helpful to you?' is also empowering since it hands over control to the lamenter. This question presents an opportunity for partnership and collaboration.

Support faith

For some, the lament is a cry to a higher power: *Hear my suffering! Get me out of here; this is such a painful place!* Clergy and chaplains are seen as messengers of God. Any human can fulfill this role, just by careful listening. Deep listening is in fact the spiritual experience some patients seem to need from their physicians. What is heard, the lament, can be reflected back in the form of a blessing, prayer, or affirmation. Listening becomes a powerful and moving experience.

Many will find comfort in reading Psalms, Job, and Lamentations, since they give voice to feelings of the sufferer.

Support the best self

Self-perception is by definition subjective. The lamenter connects with helplessness, loss, failure, and shame. Positive qualities are often forgotten and self-esteem suffers. The listener can often quite sincerely remind the lamenter of personal strengths that are being overlooked.

Introduce hope

Without negating the negative perceptions of the lamenter, the listener, through his/her spirit, positivity, humor, humanity, may stimulate some of these qualities in the person lamenting. Music, poetry, story all can lift the spirit, shift mood, optimism, and perception of the situation.

Touch

Nowadays regarded with suspicion, appropriate touch, done with great care and consciousness, can be very healing. A simple touching of the hand can mean a great deal to someone who feels isolated and estranged. Very careful listening has the same effect. Dan Bloom, Gestalt psychotherapist, states this succinctly, 'I touch by my listening' (personal communication).

Attend to the Gestalt of the medical encounter

For the patient, there is life-affirming power in the routine of the office visit. A visit to the doctor is an experience that extends far beyond the encounter alone. There is a social component to the office visit.

Utilize ritual

When losses have been openly lamented and grief has been expressed, then the time has come to move on to effective action. Recommending or assisting in creation of a ritual can help to support and facilitate this transition. More about this can be found in Chapter 15.

Utilize the power of relationship

You cannot reverse losses but you can substitute for them, at least in part, with your relationship. As the patient's lament fades, your relationship emerges more prominently into the foreground. This may not occur when the lament has been played so many times that it becomes deeply ingrained into the identity of the person.

'I am a holocaust survivor' she told me. Having some time to spare as I rounded in the hospital, I thought I would invite this 75-year-old woman to tell me more. She vividly described a harrowing journey of survival as a teenager across Eastern Europe through Turkey, Lebanon into Palestine, yet her voice was flat and monotonous. Somewhere around the Caucasus I began to have this funny feeling that I could continue on my rounds and she would continue the telling of her story regardless of my absence. Her story had been told for 40 years and she would continue with the retelling 'til she died.

Differential diagnosis

Should the lament be associated with other features of major depression, then referral to a psychiatrist or treatment with antidepressants may be indicated.

Laments frequently co-exist with or are triggered by organic illness. Diagnosing suffering does not relieve you from the responsibility of practicing good clinical medicine and ensuring that patients receive appropriate investigations and treatment.

References

1 Seeger P (1997) Housewife's lament. *Penelope Isn't Waiting Any More*. Rounder 401.1: LP.

2 Rosner F (1998) *The Medical Legacy of Moses Maimonides*. Ktav Publishing House, Jersey City, NJ.

3 Preuss J (1983) *Julius Preuss' Biblical and Talmudic Medicine*. Hebrew Publishing Company, New York.

4 Rabbi Nachman's Wisdom 50. www.breslov.org (accessed 21 June 2005) (personal communication).

5 Daugird A, Spencer D (1996) Physician reactions to the health care revolution: a grief model approach. *Arch Fam Med.* **5**: 497–500.

6   Loder D (1998) *The Saddest Day of My Life*. Berks County Medical Record, May 1998.

7   Brouillette J (1996) Physician moaning syndrome. *J Florida MA*. **83**: 139.

8   Byrne P (2002) 'Give sorrow words': lament − contemporary need for Job's old time religion. *J Pastoral Care*. **56**: 255–64.

9   Kroenke K (2003) Patients presenting with somatic complaints: epidemiology, psychiatric comorbidity and management. *Int J Methods Psychiatr Res*. **12**: 34–43.

10 Barks C (1995) *The Essential Rumi*. HarperCollins, New York.

11 Basskim L (1997) Note to doctors: stop whining (letter). *Med Econ*. **24**: 20.

12 *New York Times* (1999) The hours that make a student an MD. 21 November.

13 Bub B (2004) The patient's lament: hidden key to effective communication: how to recognise and transform. *Med Humanit*. **30**: 63–9.

14 Schneider JM (1994) *Finding My Way. Healing and Transformation through Loss and Grief*. Seasons Press, Colfax, WI.

15 Frankl VE (1946) *Man's Search for Meaning*. Beacon Press, New York.

14

What to use: *metaphor and simile*

> The physics of a man's circulation
> are the physics of the waterworks of the town
> Sir William Osler

In the preceding chapters we focused on setting the stage for healthy communication by:

- deconstructing some of the fixed images that create resistance to communication
- emphasizing self-care as an essential component of authentic communication
- discussing the creation of time and space for listening
- teaching what to listen for
- indicating some pitfalls of communication that might traumatize rather than heal
- introducing some concepts such as The Lament and The Healing Plan.

In the next few chapters we will cover some specific techniques that will aid communication. Even though these are only a select few, they will give you a taste of the tools available to you.

At a lecture relating to medical humanities, the speaker said the following:

I have been afflicted with severe Crohn's colitis my entire adult life. Relapses were occasionally life-threatening, and there was never a day when I could take my health for granted. How I envied other kids running off to college, having fun, chasing girls, living care-free lives. My career suffered, my relationships were challenged, the list goes on.

One day, after more than 20 years of the disease, I needed to see another gastroenterologist — by this stage I had seen many.

This doctor did something unique. He asked me, 'Frank, how has this disease affected your life?'

> I am not sure who was more surprised, him or me, when I burst into tears! His question had opened up a floodgate of contained grief. You see, he had touched a nerve. No doctor had ever before acknowledged my suffering.

'Touched a nerve' – imagine someone touching an exposed nerve in a tooth. Beyond sensitive, this is exquisitely painful. A nerve – like Frank's suffering – is normally protected and hidden, and the gastroenterologist's question managed to precisely locate and touch it. The use of this metaphor enabled Frank to vividly express his experience.

The physician could have followed up with a metaphor of his own: 'If you were to describe your life to me as a *something*, what would it be?'

Frank might then have been encouraged to find another metaphor as he answered *My life is a*:

- *prison*: I am shackled to physicians, medications, pharmacies and never feel free just to be me
- *roller coaster*: I never know when I my Crohn's will take a terrifying turn for the worse
- *rose garden*: it is mostly sweet with occasional thorn pricks which hurt
- *mountain*: it is mostly an uphill slog with occasional level patches.

Each metaphor offers an insight into Frank's unique perspective, one which can be amplified by another follow-up question, 'Can you describe the mountain?' or 'What is the worst part of being on a roller coaster?' Then Frank could be asked, 'What would make the climb easier for you?' or 'What would make the roller coaster more bearable?' In other words, *what do you need?*

Metaphor allows for the creation of a lively and rich dialogue. It transforms *talking about* something into *a vivid experience of* something beyond the simple transmission of facts. What it does is to stimulate the speaker to really search for the flavor or the essence of the issue, and in the process to develop new and often valuable insights as he does so.

Simile and metaphor are closely related, but, unlike metaphor, a simile uses *like* or *as*. An example might be: 'The bump on my head feels *like a ripe tomato*' or 'My belly feels bloated *like a balloon.*'

Uses of metaphor and simile

To explain complex medical concepts

They offer an alternative to professional jargon which is frequently confusing, alienating, and intimidating.

Plumbing

The patient is in shock, and it isn't clear if it is cardiogenic or related to the septicemia. How to explain to the patient's engineer son? One way is as follows, 'Imagine the cardiovascular system is like the plumbing in your house. You turn the faucet yet no water flows – the pressure is too low. The problem is either related to the pump failing, the pipes dilating or leaking, or insufficient water. In the body, the heart is the pump; blood vessels are the pipes; blood is the water in the pipes. We need to find out where the problem lies.'

To facilitate understanding and counseling

It is always best to elicit a personal metaphor or simile, since not only does this provide a more graphic image of the patient's perspective, but it also limits the practitioner from projecting a personal image that may not be as relevant. Still, there are times when it is helpful for you to offer your own. Your metaphor may reframe the issue and it may also demonstrate that you understand the nature of the situation. Depending on your area of work, you may develop metaphors that are most useful for you.

Lifestyle and well-being

Life as a pizza

A patient complains of fatigue and no physical cause has been found. The practitioner wants to demonstrate his impression that it is psychogenic – most likely related to a dysfunctional lifestyle. 'Imagine your life as a pizza,' she says. 'You can divide it up into three slices. One is your satisfaction from *WORK*; the other is your satisfaction from *PLAY*, i.e., your interests, the fun stuff you do; and the third *LOVE*, i.e., your relationships. Draw this pizza showing how large the slices of your life are.' As he divides his pizza, it becomes apparent to him that since his marriage and job are unsatisfactory, and his fun activities mediocre, that there exists a large void in the 'pizza' that is his life.

Chronic illness and resiliency

The palm tree

When I think of all the things being thrown your way, I am reminded of a palm tree. It needs to have an inner strength so that it can support itself and stand upright; it must be firmly rooted so it does not blow away; it needs to be flexible so that it bends rather than breaks; it needs to have recuperative ability to rebound after the storm. That's a lot to ask of a palm tree, isn't it? How do you see yourself?

The wave

'You are at the ocean, jumping the waves in high tide. Just when you think it's safe to relax you turn your back and a big one hits you.'

Whenever possible, be spontaneous. Use metaphors that emerge from the environment. One day I was speaking with a patient in his hospital room that faced a river. As we were talking, a tugboat pushing a barge passed into our field of view in the window. We were both distracted by it. 'Who is helping your boat move up river.' From this emerged a very useful dialogue.

Difficulty in changing behavior

We know how difficult it is to change behavior. Patients may come in feeling guilty at their lapses. The following demonstrates empathy.

The red light

'Imagine you are driving along a road that you have not been on before and you drive right through a red light without noticing it. Your partner points it out to you. The next time you are on that road you notice the red light but too late; you have already driven through it. The next time you screech to a halt just in time. The fourth time you look out for the red light and easily stop in time.'

The sail boat

'You are sailing and you need to turn the boat, so you pull on the rudder. Nothing happens, so you pull on it again. Nothing again, so this time you pull hard and the boat overcorrects almost capsizing you. Change takes time. Go easy, don't overcorrect.'

The Exodus process

Whether it is moving to a new town, promotion to a new position, beginning menopause, entering the hospital for surgery, or undergoing a divorce, transitions are at best challenging and uncomfortable, and at worst threatening and painful. They require a reorganization of self, a shift in awareness of *who I am* and *what am I becoming*. Transitions that appear positive often include hidden losses and those that are overtly painful usually have hidden gains. Not infrequently, there is nostalgia and a desire to turn back to what feels safe and comfortable. Nevertheless, change is inevitable and the individual is offered only one basic choice. *Do I resist or do I embrace change consciously so that even situations fraught with potential losses become opportunities for personal growth?*

Fortunately, the Bible offers a metaphoric roadmap in the form of the book of Exodus (*The Road Out*). In this book are to be found all the distinct stages of a journey, and these can serve to guide the patient on her travels.

The Exodus Process

She is a battered wife and needs to leave her husband, and yet is ambivalent. You refer to Exodus and ask her:

- What can be the burning bush for you? What signal do you need to begin your process of liberation?
- What are the plagues that are afflicting you?
- You remain in Egypt, avoiding the march to freedom – why?
- What is the Pharaoh, the voice of resistance, inside of you that stops you from leaving?
- You hesitate at the Red Sea. Describe your fears. What do you need to take the plunge?
- Now you are on the other side, like Miriam and her timbrels, who is there to rejoice with you?
- You are wandering in the wilderness, the journey seems very long and you want it to end. It takes time to transform identity from slave to free person. In what way were you a slave, and what needs time to die in you so that you can be truly free?
- You want to return to Egypt. You are nostalgic for the 'fleshpots'. Even slavery felt better that the uncertainty of your existence right now.
- You are angry with God for taking you away from the safety of being a slave in Egypt. You would rather die a slave than wander around without shelter. What do you want to say to God?
- God has rained manna on you. In what way have you received unexpected blessings?
- Now you are worshipping the golden calf. Freedom involves the responsibility of making good choices. It is so easy to worship false idols. What are the important values you need to retain as a free person?

- You have been given the Ten Commandments. What are the golden rules you now live your life by?
- You are entering the Promised Land. What does your Utopia look like?

The Exodus metaphor can be used in many ways for transitions that feel long and frightening, such as chronic illness, repeated surgeries, cancer treatment, etc.

In guided imagery

A simile or metaphor may open the way to healing imagery. A patient may, for example, describe searing herpes zoster pain as 'a lion scratching at my skin with his claws'. In leading a patient through a guided imagery, this lion is seen to be rather small. They probe this image of the lion further, and see that it has the qualities of a pesky pussy cat – one that can be contained in a cage. The pain does not disappear, but it is less overwhelming, and there is now less fear associated with it.

In prayer

An intravenous infusion of antibiotics is uncomfortable, disturbing, and alien, particularly when the infusion is needed for 6 weeks or more. My wife and I wrote a prayer for healing from osteomyelitis or a septic joint infection, in which we transformed intravenous fluid into 'healing dew'.

Prayer for healing

We praise the Source of Life, present in the miracle of human being, for the healing powers of body, mind, and spirit.
Grant _____ [me][him][her] ever renewing faith, courage, and comfort.
May each osteoblast, the cells which heal bones, be like the angel Gabriel, bringing strength and healing bonding.
May each white corpuscle, the cells which conquer infection, be like the angel Uriel, carrying healing light to the site of surgery, rapidly closing each wound.
May each medication be supported by Your messenger Raphael, the angel of healing. Let each droplet of medication be a healing dew for _____ [me][her][him], Your creation.

May Your presence, Holy One, light up [my][her][him] _____ 's spirit, nurturing [me][her][him] and [my][her][his] loved ones, now and forever more.
Blessed is the Healer of all flesh. Amen.
Composed by Rabbi Goldie Milgram and Dr Barry Bub

In this prayer, we created several similes:

- osteoblasts: became *like the angel Gabriel* (from Hebrew *gibor* strength)
- white corpuscle: became *like the angel Uriel* (from Hebrew *uri* light)
- medication: became *like the angel Raphael* (from Hebrew *refuah* healing).

We also created two metaphors:

- patient: became *Your Creation*
- God became: *Healer of all flesh*.

A word of caution

While similes and metaphors can heal, they can also traumatize. Obviously in poor communication, this can occur. One attractive teenager saw her dermatologist for an acne follow-up. The dermatologist noting her bangs down to her eyebrows said, 'You don't need your bangs to hide the acne, besides they make your nose look *like a ski slope*.'

It is essential that metaphors and similes be appropriate to the patient. To use the Exodus process or a prayer for healing with an atheist would clearly be a poor choice.

15

What to use: *ritual*

Much that passes for education is not education at all but ritual. The fact is that we are being educated when we know it least.

DP Gardner[1]

We live in a left-brain world where speech dominates our communication. Nevertheless, talking *about* a traumatic experience is of little healing value, for several reasons. Significant trauma does not only affect the left brain, it is frozen in the limbic system, right brain, and the entire body. In fact, memory of the trauma may well be sealed off from language.

A carefully enacted *conscious* ritual – one that encourages introspection, processing and planning; gathers together supportive community; creates space for speech and sharing of thoughts and emotions; utilizes symbols that are the metaphors of the issue; involves a whole body enactment in the here and now – is holistically healing in a way that mere talking alone can never be.

But this is not how ritual is currently being used in medicine ...

Once a week Meg, an internist, rushes off to attend a noontime lecture at the local hospital. She signs the attendance sheet, helps herself to some lunch, and settles down to listen. The sponsor, a pharmaceutical company, is thanked. The lecturer is introduced, then he steps up to the podium, offers thanks for the invitation and introduction, cracks a joke, turns down the lights, adjusts the slide projector or PowerPoint, and delivers his presentation pointing to data on the screen as he goes along.

The audience listens passively. They are, as always, seated in rows looking alternately at the screen and at the backs of the heads of those sitting in front. Some find their attention wandering and they begin to fidget or nod off.

After 45 minutes the lecture is concluded, questions are asked, the speaker is thanked, and participants hand in their evaluations at the door.

The medical lecture is a highly ritualized activity that has a distinct structure familiar to all in medical community. As is customary today, it is centered around technology – the slide projector or computer. This is an example of an *unconscious ritual*, one that is enacted without awareness of its significance. When seen this way, it becomes obvious that many unconscious rituals are enacted in the day-to-day lives of healthcare professionals.

In a typical day, Meg wakes up, orients herself, putters off to the kitchen, defrosts a bagel, turns on the coffee maker, switches on the TV to CNN, then steps outside to pick up the *New York Times*. This is her routine. It is her morning ritual.

As a family doctor she sees many people for follow-up of their hypertension. They are weighed at every visit, and, after some social chitchat, she reviews their medications, listens to their heart and lungs, takes their pulse, and checks their blood pressure. They are scheduled to return in 3 months. She has been doing this ritual for years.

She looks forward to lunch today. Every Friday, a pharmaceutical representative is scheduled to bring lunch to the office. This is an opportunity for her and the employees to relax over pizza or assorted cold sandwiches, and is a nice way to end the week. Sure, there is a brief presentation, but mostly it is an opportunity for the staff to socialize and discuss patients.

Being Friday, Meg packs the pile of journals that have accumulated over the past week into a carton and takes them home. There they will sit in her living room to await her attention during her leisure time. She and her husband have a drink. He complains about his day, she complains about hers. They have dinner and then she dozes off as she watches TV.

She somehow never finds the right time to read her journals, so they sit untouched. Feeling somewhat guilty, Meg will later move them to her study where they are less visible. Eventually these journals will migrate to the garage and, a few months later, still unread, Meg will throw them into the trash, since there are now newer journals waiting to be read.

This is all very predictable, yet she faithfully repeats this ritual week after week.

These patterns of behavior are some of Meg's routines – her rituals. They are performed pro forma and, as such, she does not have to apply conscious thought to their enactment. They provide a rhythm and structure to her life, and mostly make her feel less anxious. This is normal human behavior. They serve a useful purpose, and yet there are drawbacks – they take time and they are used in place of newer rituals that may be more meaningful and useful to her current circumstances. What would happen if Meg examined her rituals and made some changes?

- *Morning ritual.* Meg is tired of arriving grumpy to work every day. Instead of taking in the news which is almost always negative, she listens to classical music while preparing breakfast. She then spends 20 minutes on the treadmill, showers, and dresses. She arrives at work feeling centered and positive. She saves the news for Sunday when she spends a couple of leisurely hours reading the weekend edition of the *Times* over brunch. She looks forward to that.
- *Blood pressure ritual.* Meg has decided that doing a cursory examination of the heart and lungs is a waste of time since this rarely elicits any useful information. Once a year, she does a thorough physical examination instead. She uses her time during the visit very specifically to review her patients' diet, exercise, medication, weight, and blood pressure. Time saved is used for communication.
- *The luncheon ritual.* This is one ritual that she decides to keep since it serves a valuable purpose. Eating lunch together boosts morale, allows the staff to let off steam, socialize, release tension, and share information about patients. She makes some changes however, by limiting conversation about office policy and patients to the last 15 minutes after the pharmaceutical representative has left. This policy boundaries confidential information and makes the lunch more useful.
- *Journal ritual.* Why, she asks, does journal reading need to be a chore? Meg forms a journal club, and she and her colleagues meet monthly over dinner at a favorite restaurant and share highlights of articles of particular interest. An unexpected benefit has been that these meetings have become fun and a useful networking experience.
- *Homecoming ritual.* She realizes that she tends to spill negativity from her day onto her husband. Now, when she comes home, she immediately heads for a long, hot shower. As she stands under the soothing running water, she reviews the events of the day. After her shower she jots down any ideas that need action later, and then heads off to have a drink with her husband, her mind and body now refreshed.

The result of her examining her unaware rituals, bringing them to a conscious level, and transforming them, is that Meg now not only feels healthier, more fulfilled, and empowered – she is more productive and has time to spare.

What exactly is ritual?

The word *ritual* is a loose term that encompasses customary behavior that ranges from the instinctive mating behavior of insects, fish, birds, and animals – to the rites of secret societies – to religious observances – to a formalized ceremony performed with intention.

Robbie E. Davis-Floyd in 'Ritual in the hospital: giving birth the American way' describes ritual as 'a patterned, repetitive, and symbolic enactment of a cultural belief or value; its primary purpose is alignment of the belief system of the individual with society.'[2]

With the medical lecture, for example, the medical profession (society) has established norms that centers learning on technology (slide projector); confirms power on the lecturer (hierarchy); projects passivity and ignorance onto the audience (community); and dictates that learning is basically verbal and left-brained.

Most rituals in society or in medicine are enacted *unconsciously*. Wash on Mondays, shopping on Fridays, turkey on Thanksgiving – most rituals are done without any conscious intent.

Others may be *partially consciously* performed, e.g., birthdays, anniversaries, marriages, and holidays. These have an intent that is obvious – they mark transitions, though the meaning is often not thought through and expanded on. The nurses' tea break is an example that is described in one article as a time for ventilating, releasing tension, sharing, and connection.[3] The downside is that this ritual does not lead to effective protest or corrective action for aspects of the job that really need to be changed (DS Lee, personal communication, November 2004).

A third category of ritual includes ones that are *consciously* performed. Here an individual or group pauses and intentionally sets out to carefully craft a ritual that is meaningful and appropriate. A conscious ritual needs to be regularly re-evaluated lest it slip into the unconscious over time.

Specific application of ritual to medicine

Many rituals in medicine date their origin to the Florence Nightingale era and the Crimean war even though medicine and the spectrum of disease have changed enormously since those days. In an address to the University of Missouri on 26 September 1904,[4] the Surgeon-General spoke on the topic 'The Elimination of Disease.' He referred to cholera, yellow fever, bubonic plague, smallpox, tuberculosis, typhoid fever, measles, scarlet fever, malarial fever, and diphtheria. He made no mention of coronary artery disease, cancer, and depression. Despite the vast disparity between pathology of past and present, rituals have mostly been adapted not consciously revised. As a result, the medical literature is generally critical of ritual:

> The term 'ritual' is often used in a pejorative sense in nursing literature to refer to unthinking, routinized action by nurses, which lacks any empirical foundation.[5]

And:

> Attitudes have changed drastically over the centuries towards people with infections and how to contain them. Only as we approach the end of the 20th century are we starting to base our practices on scientific evidence and not on ritual, although rational thought is still not found in many practices, and confusion surrounds the terminology used.[6]

Yes, ritual is often 'unthinking routinized action,' and yes, 'rational thought' is frequently not found in many practices, and yet even unconscious ritual often serves a useful function. It creates a structure that lessens anxiety, offers meaning, and bonds society. Doing things as a society in a routinized way creates familiarity and safety. There are other rituals that are not routine and they serve another function, which is healing.

Many rituals are described in great length in the Bible. The ancients used ritual, incense, and music in their healing rituals. Shamans, medicine men, witchdoctors have utilized ritual since time immemorial. Only in modern medicine have we avoided using the power that ritual offers, even though we are aware that many of the issues that distress patients involve change of status, e.g., loss of health, miscarriage, menopause, surgery. Many fears and feelings are not totally rational, and the medium we use to communicate in medicine – verbal, rational discourse – is just not enough; in fact it is irrational to expect that it would be!

Once the medical profession revises its attitude to ritual, then the profession can begin to tap the enormous healing power that ritual offers. It requires a two-step approach that involves:

1   critically examining practices and rituals, and discarding those that are simple hold-overs from an earlier time in favor of new behaviors that are more efficient and meaningful to present circumstances
2   creating conscious rituals that support personal and professional growth, communication, change, and healing.

The utilization of conscious ritual

Rituals are most useful when they accompany transitions, particularly major life transitions. In general, these fall into five functional categories.

1 *Beginnings*: birth, graduation, new job, onset of chemotherapy, surgery, etc.
2 *Mergings*: marriage, partnership, etc.
3 *Cycles*: anniversaries, holidays, birthdays, etc.
4 *Endings*: end of treatment, menopause, retirement, etc.
5 *Healings*: recovery from illness and trauma etc.

Each transition or rite of passage represents an opportunity for a ritual to deepen and enrich the significance of the change of status of the individual and society. There are also more minor transitions like entering the workplace or returning home from a day's work. They too can benefit from conscious ritual as Meg noticed.

Conscious rituals have much to offer. They:

- acknowledge the meaning and significance of the transition
- enact a belief system to be embodied by the participants
- provide the framework of support for change
- allow for identification of losses and gains inherent in all transitions
- affirm the identity of the individual and his/her place in community
- provide a context for the event within the larger picture
- transform the transition into spiritual experience
- support the emerging identity of the person and/or community
- support the family and community of the person in transition
- facilitate celebration or mourning
- promote healing.

A good example of the possible use of ritual might be the woman who is about to have a total hysterectomy. This will make her menopausal – a significant life transition. In a classic three-stage rite of passage, the patient will:

1 separate from her community as she enters the hospital
2 go through the liminal (transitional) stage of hospitalization and surgery in which she undergoes transformation
3 return to her community of family and friends very different than when she left.

What rituals help her through this?

The present-day unconscious ritual involves all the elements of a typical hospitalization – insurance information, wrist band, intake with history, bowel prep, etc. The night before surgery she will be given television to watch and perhaps a sleeping pill. Her homecoming will involve some help with activities of daily living, and friends sending cards or flowers and perhaps calling.

Alternatively, she might choose to plan a conscious ritual. Prior to surgery, she would bring together friends who have already experienced the menopause. She prepares a personal statement to read aloud, selects a symbol that represents her feelings about losing her uterus and ovaries, and creates a suitable environment for the enactment. In the ritual she express her fears and emotions regarding surgery and her pending losses, and in turn receives nurturing feedback and pearls of wisdom from those who have been through the procedure. Out of this ritual might emerge awareness of hidden gains. Her friends might present her with a token of their support, perhaps a quilt embroidered with sayings, or book of poems – something that will sustain and support her through the surgery. This would be very comforting, certainly more so than watching television the night before.

Other examples of conscious ritual in medicine

Miscarriage or stillbirth

Usually a pregnancy results in a celebratory homecoming and naming ritual. With miscarriage or stillbirth there is only grief experienced alone or as a couple. The sensitive practitioner may want to inquire about a ritual to acknowledge the loss not only to the mother, but also to the father, grandparents, and siblings.

A ritual can include naming the child; letters to the child expressing their dashed hopes and feelings; the lighting of a candle; the planting of a memorial garden; the enactment of a burial ritual that involves ultrasound images and other memorabilia; the dedication of a project or selection of a charity for donations.

> The most effective rituals will come from the patient's own personal history, beliefs, culture, values, and experience. For example, to one person a candle may be meaningful, to another a candle may not be. People from different cultures and society may have their own mourning rituals that they would want to incorporate (B Yasgur, personal communication, 2004).

The practitioner need not be involved in the ritual; merely suggesting one both transmits empathy to the patient and plants an idea that may be useful. Furthermore, the practitioner may offer some assistance in the planning phase.

Infertility

Embarking on the route of infertility testing, artificial insemination, or in vitro fertilization is a major and stressful undertaking as this couple found out. In their case, it included many setbacks, a difficult pregnancy, and a caesarian section, but they were sustained by this ritual.

They recently discovered that he was infertile, and she would need artificial insemination from an anonymous donor if she wished to become pregnant. They wanted a baby created with love, and found instead that their contact with the medical environment was 'sterile', devoid of any spirit or warmth. They asked for help in preparing a ritual.

During the ritual, he wept at the thought of never fathering a child of his own. Still, his hope was to be a role model for the child. She expressed her deep love and appreciation for him, and reminded him that regardless of the biological process involved, he would be no less of a real father to their children.

She held up an empty goblet which he filled with white wine, a symbol of vitality and male energy. They both drank from it. Those present offered blessings to the couple and to their future lives as parents, and then withdrew to allow them to savor this intimate, holy time together.

Death of a patient

A ritual allows for the expression of individual feelings, builds community in the office, and affirms the 'holy' nature of the work.

- *Old ritual.* Receptionist reads of the death of a patient in the obituary section of the local newspaper (which she faithfully reads every day). The obituary notice is attached to the chart and placed on the desk by the receptionist. The physician reviews the chart and instructs that it be filed in storage, the patient's appointment be erased, and that a card be mailed to the family.
- *New ritual.* On notification of the death of a patient, a brief memorial service is held in the office. Each participant shares a memory of the patient, and then a short scripted prayer is read which gives thanks 'for the privilege of having been on the journey with this patient if only for a short period.' A card is signed by all present, and a condolence card is mailed to the spouse or closest living relative. This need only take 10 minutes.

Practice points

- Explore your routines. Which are rituals that can be discarded or modified to save you time and energy?
- Create specific rituals that enhance your well-being and spirit as you transition from waking up to entering the workplace. Likewise create rituals that allow you to detoxify from stresses and traumas at work as you arrive home. Be creative and flout convention.
- Whenever patients experience major loss or transition of any type, consider suggesting a ritual. Not everyone is open to this, but for the occasional patient that is, this suggestion can set in motion a very important healing process.
- There are very specific guidelines for creating a ritual. These involve mainly the steps in planning and enactment of one. Further information can be found on www.processmedicine.com.

References

1   Gardner DP (1975) President, University of Utah, Salt Lake. *Vital Speeches*. 15 April 1975.

2   Grimes R (ed) (1996) *Readings in Ritual Studies*, pp. 146–58. Prentice Hall, Upper Saddle River, NJ.

3   Lee DST (2001) The morning tea break ritual: a case study. *Int J Nurs Pract*. **7**: 69–73.

4   Reiling J (2004) JAMA 100 years ago: the elimination of disease. *JAMA*. **292**: 2288.

5   Philpin SM (2002) Rituals and nursing: a critical commentary. *J Adv Nurs*. **38**: 144–51.

6   Parker LJ (1999) Current recommendations for isolation practices in nursing. *Br J Nurs*. **8**: 881–7.

16

What to attend to: *boundaries*

All real living is meeting
Martin Buber[1]

We try to hear and understand what is being communicated. We try to craft our words so that we respond in the most effective way possible. Nevertheless, success or failure in our communication experiences is often determined long before anyone has spoken. Our willingness to fully reveal ourselves to others is largely based on how a vital part of ourselves – one that cannot be seen, touched, or examined – is treated.

John Smith, a 56-year-old, a quiet, somewhat shy, English high-school teacher, has a few problems so he visits a local physician. This is his first visit, so he is somewhat tentative.

He enters the office and walks up to the counter. The receptionist checks his name off her list and thrusts a pen and clipboard into his hand with instructions to *complete this.*

He finds an open seat next to a woman who looks suspiciously like the mother of one of his students. He sighs and thinks this can't be helped. He turns to the form. Impersonal and to the point, he notes, probably purchased from a catalog. He begins to check off answers. What's this he wonders, *bowel habits, sexual orientation, HIV status, isn't this a little intimate especially since I haven't met the man yet?* He notices that the mother is glancing at his responses so he shields the paper from her.

Once he has finished filling out the form, he looks around and takes note of his surroundings. *Wish they would change that radio station; that pop music is really annoying,* he thinks to himself. He reaches over to pick up some reading material, *Vegetarian Monthly, Nutrition, Marathon Running* – the doctor's orientation is obvious.

'John Smith' the nurse calls out from the door leading to the hallway. On the way to the examination room she weighs and measures him. He has always been self-conscious about his weight and tries not to look down at the scale. '184 pounds, John, a little on the high side,' she comments. Noting he has a urinary problem, she hands him a cup and asks him to void into it, then get undressed and wait for the doctor in the examination room.

After 15 minutes, the doctor enters the room rattling dictation into a little recorder with machine-gun rapidity. He is accompanied by a young woman in an oversized white coat who he introduces as a medical student. He fires off a few questions, performs a brief examination, and offers reassurance. He has already begun dictation as he walks out of the office. John Smith has decided not to tell him his real reason for visiting — his promise to his wife that he would speak to a physician about his sluggish sex drive.

It's quite magical really. Each and every one of us is surrounded by an invisible bubble that is as much part of us as is our skin. It travels with us wherever we go. It is vibrant, alive, dynamic, constantly adapting and modifying itself to our inner and outer environments. In an instant, without any conscious attention on our part, this bubble can expand or contract, open or close its portals, as the situation dictates. Any shift in our sense of power, safety, trust, intimacy to others around us, and this bubble adjusts immediately and automatically. Not only attuned to our inner worlds, this bubble senses the bubbles of others who come near us. It senses and interprets the signals that are being sent to us, and informs us on the signals we need to send in turn to ensure our safety. We modify our behavior, voice, dress, gesture, touch, movement, accordingly. Like dogs peeing on poles and water hydrants, we place objects in areas of our personal territory such as seat, desk, or room that indicate THIS IS MY ROOM/SPACE KEEP OUT! The way we arrange our appearance, behavior, and environment tells others the state of our bubble.

Our bodies are designed to facilitate the sending of signals to others. Our many facial muscles, and the fact that much of our face is bare of hair, help us to do that. In turn, we have the ability to read subtle messages of others, distinguishing between natural laughter and forced laughter, natural smiles and forced ones, honest spontaneous responses and ones that are not.

Inside this bubble is our intimate space into which we only invite people to whom we feel very close. Their bubbles make way for ours, and our bubbles merge enclosing us in an intimate cocoon of relationship. My wife and I call it our 'cave'.

Radiating out from this intimate space are circles of space sequentially allocated to friendship, social contacts, and to public impersonal contacts.

Hall explored humans' perception and use of space, and in 1959 he labeled this study of space *proxemics*.[2] He described the appropriate physical distances between people in various relationships.

- Intimate: 0–18 inches.
- Personal: 18 inches to 4 feet.
- Social: 4–10 feet.
- Public: greater than 10 feet.

This bubble regulates our every behavior in society; the way we stand in elevators; the seat we choose in a restaurant, library, or park bench; where we choose to place our brief cases when we sit down; our choice of clothing, words, and gestures that signal our relationship to the outside world. It separates us from others, giving us and others a feeling of individuality and psychological and physical safety.

Many factors influence our bubble, including cultural and societal norms, age, gender, relationship, and history of previous trauma. Every encounter and relationship creates a shift – waitress, shop assistant, spouse, patient, stranger on bus, child – each one creates an immediate alteration in shape and porousness of this bubble.

This bubble or boundary space or interpersonal boundary generates such deeply rooted, unconscious, instinctive behavior that it must be important and indeed it is. Our greatest traumas occur when our boundaries are violated.

Since our boundaries protect us and maintain our identity in a changing environment, what happens to them when we cross the threshold from sidewalk to medical office, and are instantly transformed in our identity from being a citizen such as John Smith *teacher* to John Smith *patient*?

To understand this it is helpful to imagine a world without interpersonal boundaries, a world where it is be normal for someone to walk into your home, use your toothbrush, and read your mail; where someone at the table next to yours in a restaurant reaches over and takes your chicken leg; where a stranger approaches you to comment on your haircut. This doesn't generally happen because of interpersonal boundaries. But there are exceptions, a doctor's office for example, a place where you can be asked the most personal questions and be touched in the most private places by a total stranger.

Fairy tales take us to imaginary worlds and yes, indeed, there is one that describes a world without boundaries:

Once upon a time, there lived a little girl named Goldilocks. She went for a walk in the forest and came upon a house and she knocked ... Sadly, our pretty little heroine was a boundary violator. She entered the family Bears' house uninvited; she sat on their chairs breaking one in the process, she ate their food, she lay on their beds, and then ran away when the owners returned. Goldilocks invaded their space and even damaged their property. She showed no respect for the boundaries of others. The Bears, victims in this story, felt transgressed upon. It wasn't so much the material damage, as the feeling that someone had violated their private personal space. Since then, feeling less secure, they regularly engaged in rituals such as locking their doors and checking that their windows were shut tight whenever they left the house. When they returned home, the first thing Papa Bear would then do was a quick tour to make sure that nobody had intruded.

We are mostly unconscious of boundaries except when they are intruded upon. Then we experience a 'felt sense'[3] that something in our bodily perception just doesn't feel right – someone being overly familiar, our seat at a conference being taken by another, a neighbor borrowing our tool kit without permission, etc. You will also notice this 'felt sense' if someone stands too close to you. The distance that feels comfortable is measurable and very specific.

John Smith had this feeling. It was as if all his boundaries so carefully cultivated outside his doctor's office had suddenly been stripped away and now he felt vulnerable and exposed.

Since the boundary space of bubble is essentially protective, the greater the feeling of *power*, the greater the sense of *safety*, the more open and relaxed the *boundary* can be.

As a patient, John felt powerless and exposed. Had an effort been made to develop a rapport with him, he might have felt more trusting, less vulnerable, and he might have shared his concerns.

This inverse relationship between trust, power, etc., and boundaries can be viewed as an equation:

Trust + Power + Safety = The extent to which boundaries can relax.

When trust, power and safety are enhanced, then communication is facilitated.

'It's my nerves, Doc,' Dorothy whined. 'I can't sleep, I feel edgy and jumpy. My skin has that crawly, itchy feeling, like insects running up and down it, and I can't sit still and nothing seems to help, what I can do to relax?' Dorothy was a spry 78-year-old woman who looked younger than her age. Harry, her husband, too complained of 'bad nerves' that he attributed to arthritis of his neck and poor vision. Dorothy blamed much of her problem on her relationship with Harry. With few friends, few interests, no children, they had little in common other than their long morning walks and their respective problems with 'bad nerves'.

No way would Dorothy see a psychotherapist at her stage of life. 'I'm too old, Doc. I just have to accept my life the way it is.' Anxiety attacks had her rushing to the emergency room at least once a year. A psychiatrist was consulted: *adjustment reaction with anxious mood*, he pronounced. He adjusted her medication, but bouts of anxiety and depression continued to plague her – and consequently me, since there was nothing I could do for her.

One day, Dorothy surprised me with something other than a *kvetch*. Less complaining, she seemed genuinely upset. 'It's been an awful week,' she sniffed into her lace handkerchief, 'My sister died. She was the last of my four siblings. I should have spent more time with her. Now she's gone too. She was very different from me. She, *sniff*, knew how to have fun. She was married, had children and friends. I used to envy her.'

Dorothy dried her eyes. 'I'll be all right,' she said. I was intrigued, however. Could it be that all the talk *about* her nerves was really a deflection from her real issues? Perhaps here was an opportunity to learn more. I suggested she return the following week and that she bring along a photo of her sister.

One week later, Dorothy was all smiles. 'My nerves are better, Doc. My nephews have been so very nice. The funeral went well. I'm OK now.'

'I'm pleased to hear that. Do you have the photo?' I asked nevertheless.

The photograph had been carefully wrapped in a silk scarf which she peeled back to reveal a gold-framed 8 by 10 benign-looking older version of herself, but with a warm smile and fewer worry lines. Taking the photograph, I placed it on the desk facing her.

'I feel much better, Doc. I'm definitely getting over it,' she insisted.

Positioning myself to the side and slightly behind her, I gently suggested, 'Why don't you tell Mary how you feel.'

At this, Dorothy burst into an avalanche of tears and deep sobs. I gently touched her shoulder and allowed her to cry. I had never seen her like this before. Finally, her crying and heaving settled down. Between the sobs, she started to speak.

'Mary, I feel so bad that I didn't spend more time with you, instead I worried about my own problems and now, now you're gone.'

With some encouragement, she continued, 'You know, I used to be jealous of you, you having so much. But I loved you and I should have called more often.' She spoke some more, mainly about old times, then gradually calmed down, and the sobbing and the words died down. She just sat there with all her emotions seemingly drained away.

'Dorothy,' I asked very softly, 'what is it you need?'

Quite suddenly, she stiffened and forcefully spat out 'Everyone is being so kind but they keep on telling me I'll be OK but that's not what I want! No one comes near me! I wish someone would give me a hug! I feel so alone!' Now she was crying again.

Oh, dear, what do I do? I thought.

'Dorothy, I'd be honored if you let me hug you.'

'You would, you really would? You're my doctor ... you would hug me?'

As she cleaved to me, I could feel her sobs against my chest – a disorienting and intensely intimate experience. After a while, she separated herself from me, dried her eyes, blew her nose, and we both sat down.

Now quite calm, she looked directly at me and said, 'You know Harry and I have no physical contact. Even when there is a particularly nasty lightning storm and I'm scared and get into his bed, he just rolls over and pulls the blankets over himself. We haven't touched for years. No one touches me. It is a painfully lonely experience.'

At a later visit she was to observe, 'I see now that Harry is limited. He just can't help himself. It's OK to want companionship. I'm not crazy for wanting it.'

As far as I know, Dorothy never again had to rush to the ER with an attack of 'nerves'.

By asking her (rather than telling her) what she needed, I offered her power. I then, with awareness, stretched boundaries and hugged her, having taken care to ask her permission first.

Having made the point that boundary space is like a bubble that separates and protects identity, I now need to confess that this is not really true. A bubble would isolate. A personal boundary not only separates and protects identity, it is also a place of meeting where identity is created. Just as light is both a particle and a wave, a boundary is both a barrier and an energy field that generates identity.

Richard Hycner, quoting the philosopher Martin Buber, wrote: 'The inter-human is that realm by which we are both separate, and in-relation. We are as much *a-part-of*, as well *as apart from*, other human beings.'[4]

> If I am I, because I am I,
> and you are you because you are you,
> then I am I and you are you.
> But if I am I because you are you,
> and if you are you because I am I,
> then I am not I, and you are not you.
>
> (Hasidic quote)

This brain-twister ancient Hasidic wisdom quoted above refers to the fact that identity is formed from the encounter of one from the other at the contact boundary. Who we are is shaped by our contact with our environment and those who are in it.

In the doctor–patient relationship, the identity of each is modified and formed by the other. If for no other reason, this limits the practitioner from being an objective observer. Professionalism requires that this be understood and integrated into the relationship.

Healthy boundaries are dynamic, fluid, and flexible. They adjust seamlessly from social, to personal, to intimate as the nature of the relationship changes. They are also semi-permeable, filtering what the individual is willing to take in or transmit to others. A useful comparison is to a house, the windows of which can be open or shut depending on the season.

Unhealthy boundaries are fixed, rigid and either wide open or tightly shut. Here the house has windows that are either always shut or always open.

One day, I asked my class of clergy students the following question: 'Occasionally you need to speak privately to a child from your Sunday school class, right? You meet in your office. Where do you ask the child to sit?'

One student gestured to a distant spot in the room at the door and was quite emphatic: 'As far away from me as possible.' Another said, 'Close by, sometimes on my lap, and I always give the child a hug.'

Each of these two students staked out an extreme position to which each rigidly adhered to *regardless of the relationship or needs of the child.* The one distanced the child; the other invaded its boundaries.

Problematic boundaries may occur with personality disorders which are commonly encountered in primary care.[5] Issues also arise with trauma victims.

- A core manifestation of Borderline Personality Disorder is the demonstration of unstable boundaries. Key to management of patients with borderline personality is the creation and adherence to very clear, firm boundaries.
- Patients with schizoid personality disorder may need a significantly greater physical and emotional distance in order to feel safe. They tend to be withdrawn, isolated, aloof, and distant, and feel easily invaded by others. You need to be very sensitive to this, since normal warmth and friendliness on your part may feel unsafe and send this person fleeing.
- Patients who have been severely traumatized sexually and otherwise may have rigid, closed boundaries. Their bubbles have turned into body armor. These boundaries need to be carefully respected as well. Some may have been traumatized by the healthcare system, and you will need to be patient and sensitive if you are to gain their trust.
- Boundaries may be excessively leaky or porous. A physician who is suffering from reimbursement woes may spill his lament to a pharmaceutical representative. A patient whose marriage is floundering may unconsciously signal sexual neediness, vulnerability, availability to the physician or vice versa, and the consequences are predictable.

Practice points

- Take note of the signals you are unwittingly sending to others regarding your boundaries. Become conscious of them and modify them if necessary. Set the tone that while you are warm and friendly, yours remains a professional relationship. Highly visible photos of your children and spouse are helpful.
- If you are going through a difficult time in your personal relationship, seek therapy if necessary. Without a safe release, it is easy to become 'leaky' and to send signals that you are in need of comfort and relationship.
- Value the sanctity of your boundaries. Establish clear boundaries and do not tolerate or signal that you will tolerate transgressions on your boundaries by others.
- Be sensitive to the boundaries of your patients being attentive to them so that they can develop trust in you. If in doubt, always ask rather than assume.

- Only when you are firmly grounded in boundaries can you then begin to stretch beyond boundaries with safety in order to create healing experiences such as described in my encounter with Dorothy.
- When afraid, patients become particularly sensitive to seemingly small details that threaten their personal space. Attend to their privacy, and avoid humor and language that signals familiarity.
- Welcome patients' families or spouses since the support they provide allows your patients to be less fearful and guarded.

References

1   Buber M (1923) *I and Thou* (RG Smith, translation). Charles Scribner and Sons, New York.

2   Hall E (1973) *The Silent Language*. Anchor Books Doubleday, New York (reissue).

3   Gendlin E (1982) *Focusing* (2e). Bantam, New York.

4   Hycner R (1991) *Between Person and Person. Toward a Dialogical Psychotherapy*, p. 7. Gestalt Journal Press, Highland, New York.

5   Hueston W, Werth J, Mainous A (1999) Personality disorder traits: prevalence and effects on health status in primary care patients. *Int J Psychiatry Med.* **29**: 63–74.

17

What to use:
psychotherapy

We can grasp nothing except through our experience[1]

Spagnuolo Lobb

Just your ability to listen empathetically will add a significant and satisfying dimension to your practice. And yet, there are times when this is not enough, since much that you are listening to comes from an unconscious, unaware place. You grapple for techniques to reveal and illuminate the real issue, the one behind the words – i.e., the story behind the story; the emotion behind the emotion. Psychological issues are almost never what they seem. You search for the means to raise the speaker's awareness of his or her shadow side, the one that is hidden and inaccessible without assistance. You hear strong emotions expressed, and you know that these are superficial ones; that beneath the anger lays a deep pool of sadness. You wonder, how do I respond so that we can break loose from the torrent of words – words that obscure rather than reveal? How do I assist my patients in experiencing the link between their physical symptoms and their underlying emotional issues so they may find relief?

Inevitably you will come to the same conclusion that I did – that empathy and compassion are not enough. There are real professional listening and psychotherapy skills that need to be acquired if one is to shift gears from skilled amateur to competent professional. The ones that radically shifted my awareness and insight were Focusing and Gestalt.

Focusing is a valuable aid to accessing emotions and relating them to the issues at hand. Rather than asking oneself *how or what do I feel*, (a thinking process) one checks one's body to notice directly how emotions manifest there.

Gestalt, which also fully attends to body awareness, adds another dimension to this process. It provides additional theory and awareness-raising techniques that enable the practitioner to make meaning of what is being communicated, and to help the patient or client shift perspective and behavior.

Focusing

In the 1960s, Professor Eugene Gendlin at the University of Chicago videotaped and studied hundreds of psychotherapy sessions with the aim of finding out why psychotherapy was helpful for some and not for others.

What he found was surprising. Success was based on the clients' tendency to slow down their talk and search for words to describe a feeling in their bodies. The ones who failed remained verbal, articulate, analytical, and 'in their heads'.

He then published a best-selling book in 1978, which he called *Focusing*.[2] In it he described the process that made the difference between successful and unsuccessful therapy. This book became a best seller and spawned a Focusing Institute[3] with training programs around the world.

Focusing has also found a myriad of applications based on the focuser's enhanced ability to pay attention to what is occurring naturally in the body. This can be done alone, and for seasoned practitioners it becomes a way of life; or it can be done in a partnership arrangement between a Focuser and a Listener.

Ann Weiser Cornell, PhD, describes Focusing as follows: 'Focusing is the process of listening to your body in a gentle, accepting way and hearing the messages that your inner self is sending you.'[4]

In this technique, the individual focuses on one or more vague sensations experienced in the body, for example a tightness in the neck, a lump in the throat, a pressure in the chest or upper abdomen.

This sensation, at first often quite vague, is called a *felt sense*. When carefully attended to and explored, this *felt sense* provides an entry way into the underlying emotions that cause it.

When the Focuser adopts a respectful, curious, non-judgmental, and welcoming approach to these sensations, then they provide clear direction to effective action, and then melt away since they no longer need to broadcast their message. Tension, anxiety, pressure are replaced with calmness.

Susan, a surgeon, arrives at her office filled with agitation after having had an argument with her spouse. Rather than tolerating or suppressing this feeling she spends a few minutes in her parked car Focusing. She closes her eyes, centers herself bringing her awareness from her extremities into the centre of her body, and asks herself, *What is most important right now?* She notices a vague sensation of discomfort in her chest and says, *Hello, I sense you are there, I'd like be silent for a while and keep you company.* As she deepens her contact with the felt sense, some descriptive words emerge — it feels like a fierce anger, she notes. Then she asks herself if she can support herself with this feeling and its relationship to her issue, her fight with her husband. She says *yes* and then notices that there is the 'inner critic' that says she should not feel this way. She stays with the critic, explores it, supports it, and thanks it, then returns to the felt sense in her chest, noticing that this feeling has now left. She asks if there is anything else, and since she does not notice any other sensation, thanks herself and proceeds to leave the car to enter her office, now with equanimity.

Focusing can be done anywhere. Prior to entering an examination or hospital room for example, you can pause, notice what is in your body, attend to it, and in this way be fully present to the patient. It need take only seconds.

Patients who are excited, distraught, or having difficulty making a decision can be guided through a Focusing experience to become aware of their emotions and how they relate to their decisions.

During an encounter, when you are asked a question, rather than offering a knee-jerk response, you might pause to do a brief Focusing to sense how you feel as well as think.

The major value of Focusing in medicine is that it requires a process which runs totally counter to the prevailing culture of rushing and multitasking. It requires the Focuser to slow down; center on the body (not just the thoughts); create space for emotions to emerge; welcome emotions (not judge them); empathize with having these emotions (not be critical — or, if so, to attend to the 'critic'); to be curious of complex emotions (rather than only the most superficial ones.) A major advantage is that no training in psychotherapy is needed, and that Focusing can be done alone or with a partner.

I had a powerful Focusing experience when a former patient called me to say he was going to commit suicide. Rather than respond immediately, I asked for a few minutes to absorb this rather profound request. As I Focused, a feeling of sadness emerged, and I responded, 'I don't plan to try to talk you out of whatever decision you make, and I need you to know that I feel really sad hearing you say this.' This opened up a dialogue that was to save his life. Later I was to do a formal Focusing session with a partner on the issue of my initial reaction to the suicide request, and layer by layer 15 other emotions emerged, including frustration, guilt, helplessness, anger.

Brief *Mini-Focusing* sessions are invaluable for creating a deeper listening experience.[5] When one does a lengthier Focusing, e.g., an hour-long telephone session with a partner, then the initial step is to make oneself comfortable, relax, close one's eyes, and then proceed with the four stages described by Ann Weiser Cornell:

1   Coming in − bringing awareness into your body.
2   Making contact − with something inside.
3   Deepening contact − keeping something company.
4   Coming out − bringing the session to a close.[4]

Training in Focusing is given by her and other Focusing instructors who can be located on the Focusing Institute website www.focusing.org.

Gestalt

Although others were involved, Fritz Perls was the major innovator of Gestalt psychotherapy. He and his wife Laura wrote *Ego, Hunger and Aggression*[6] in South Africa in 1942, then after the war, they moved to the USA and established the New York Gestalt Institute of which I am a member. Paul Goodman was the principal author of *Gestalt Therapy: excitement and growth in the human personality*,[7] which remains the 'bible' of Gestalt theory today. Later, Fritz was to move to the West Coast, while Laura remained in New York City − each to pursue their distinctive approach to Gestalt.

Gestalt introduced a radical shift from the Freudian model based on the intra-psychic analysis of the individual client, to the *encounter* between client and therapist, hence utilizing the healing power of relationship.

In Gestalt, emphasis is on the 'here and now'. When the past is referred to, it is only with respect to how it informs on the situation in the present.

Gestalt is also uniquely holistic. Since mind and body are inseparable, a practitioner may just as easily focus on a word, a phrase, a shrug, a hand movement, etc. to raise awareness about the state of mind of the individual.

One of the most sought-after experiences that Gestalt therapy can provide is the 'Aha!' − the sudden insight which illuminates that which was previously unseen and not understood about the self.[8] The role of the therapist is not to analyze or inform, rather it is to provide support and raise awareness so the patient has these 'Aha!' experiences.

Emphasis is on supporting healthy process − is the client or patient able to make good *contact*, or are there issues of *resistance* that create fixed images and interrupt healthy contact with the environment?

There is a significant body of theory that informs the practitioner on boundary, contact, awareness, self, organismic self-regulation, etc. This theory can be readily learned. The major challenge is for the practitioner to slow down the interaction, notice subtleties of language and movement, reflect back these observations in a way that enhances insight, and be willing to take risk in creatively setting up experiments.

The *experiment* is the cornerstone of experiential learning. 'It transforms talking about and stale reminiscing and theorizing into being fully here with all one's imagination, energy and excitement and action' (Dan Bloom, personal communication).

My pillow fight with a patient described in an earlier chapter is a classic Gestalt experiment. Many experiments are surprisingly subtle yet the 'Aha's' they produce and emotions they trigger are often remarkably powerful.

A physician client says, 'I cannot meet with my colleagues, I have to work.' My response might be, 'Try changing your language to one of empowerment, e.g., "Though I would like to go *I choose* not to join my colleagues at the meeting since *I choose* to see my patients then." What do you experience when you say this?'

Here is another experiment, one that involves dialogue between patient and an absent (in this case dead) person.

Sam had neck and upper back pain, less so when working his small garden plot than when he rested and 'thought about things'. I thought I knew him quite well, after all he and his wife had been patients for years. (How often do we make that error?) His pain could be explained by the extensive osteoarthritis of his cervical spine, but something about his story suggested that there might be another cause.

'What do you think about when you rest up?' I asked. Vague at first, he eventually began to speak about his 28-year-old stepson's suicide.

'Five years ago my stepson shot himself in his head after an argument with his wife. His mother was devastated when she discovered his body. You can't believe the mess. Since then, my wife and I have been actively participating in a survivors' support group. But you know that, right?'

No, I didn't. This was news to me.

'We are over his death now,' he said. 'The support group is mainly an important part of our social network.'

'Do you have a photograph of your stepson?' I asked. He pulled out his wallet and showed me.

'I'd like to hear you speak directly to him; tell him that you are over his death now.'

As he looked at the photograph he flushed, his forehead creased, and he began to cry. As he composed himself, he became angry.

'How could you do this to your mother, didn't you know it would ruin her life? How selfish could anyone be!' he cried as he clutched his neck which had begun to hurt.

Five years in the support group may have helped his social life but they had done remarkably little to heal his wounds.

Once having acquired some professional therapy skills, like me, you will soon find yourself chomping at the bit when you encounter a drama played out superficially while an ocean-depth of emotions, trauma, and wounding lies unexplored beneath the surface. This was my experience during a listening exercise at a conference on complementary medicine. Our instructions were to split into groups of three, with each participant taking a 5-minute turn to talk. The other two were, in the meantime, to listen without comment.

> 'I came here primarily to learn about alternative medicine,' the 40-something internist said. 'My wife has cancer and I'm here looking for something to help her. Also, it can come in useful in my practice. I'm a fallen Catholic, by the way. It doesn't bother me. I'm not religious, and in fact being neutral about religion actually helps me in my practice. I don't steer my patients in any direction. I'm a blank slate.'

A 'blank slate'? A 'fallen' Catholic who is 'neutral' about religion? A caregiver who speaks dispassionately about finding treatments for his wife's cancer, yet demonstrates minimal insight into himself and his needs. These are fixed images just begging to be challenged. Psychotherapy skills enable the listener to hear beyond the utterances.

Now it was the pediatrician's turn to speak. Attractive, in her early thirties, quite tense, her speech was rapid, and her sentences seem to run into each other without a pause.

> 'I graduated at this institution 5 years ago ... I can't believe they are actually doing a conference on healing and alternative medicine here ... There was nothing like this before ... I am having difficulty with my mothers ... wanting antibiotics for their kids with virus infections so they can return them to daycare the next day and when I say that there is little I can do they leave the office unhappy ... I am thinking of leaving to do academic medicine ... but I think maybe there is something I can learn here that could be useful ... I think it I may just have to move on ... I think practice will always be a challenge.'

Here too, midst all these words, was an outpouring of unexamined issues. All this 'thinking' – where is the *feeling-self*? All these losses – power, control, meaning, validation, support – has she actually paused long enough to listen to her feelings?

With patients, too, listening becomes much easier when one understands the mindbody connection and has some psychotherapy techniques at one's disposal.

Judy woke up one night with a choking feeling in her throat. She rushed off to the emergency room in a panic, but nothing abnormal was found. She continued to have symptoms even though all her studies were negative.

'What do you think?' she asked me.

'Our throat muscles can tighten up when we are under stress; has anything been bothering you lately?' I asked her in turn.

'Just something with my daughter. She had an abortion against my wishes and I was quite upset. Now that you mention it, my symptoms did start about then.'

I suggested that we use the *empty chair* technique in which she would talk to her daughter as if she were present in the room. She agreed to do this, and I pulled up a chair to face her.

'Imagine your daughter is sitting in front of you right now; what do you need to say to her?'

Judy became quite livid and the words spewed out. Almost immediately her throat tightened, effectively preventing her from saying things that could be difficult for her to express. Her conflict was obvious – on the one hand she wanted to chastise her daughter, and on the other hand she wanted to avoid saying anything that would drive her away.

Certainly, psychotherapy and therapeutic interventions such as these may take longer than the usual office visit, but they have a plus side.

- They reduce the need for repeat office visits.
- Most of the time, psychotherapy is useful more to deepen the practitioner's understanding of the patient's emotional state than it is to create a direct intervention such as described above. This saves time.
- Holistic medicine cannot exist without understanding of a vital dimension of the patient – the psyche. With the use of psychotherapy in mainstream medical practice, medical care becomes truly holistic.
- The alternative approach of referring the patient to 'mental health' usually requires a wait of weeks for an appointment, and further weeks or months to establish rapport between therapist and patient. With a trusting relationship already cultivated, it takes very little work on your part for a transformative experience to occur.
- Medical practice becomes fascinating, meaningful, and healing.

Practice points

There are many psychotherapeutic approaches. I favor Focusing and Gestalt in that they are holistic, firmly grounded in solid theory, and highly applicable to medical practice as brief therapy. Your choice will no doubt be based on the available training program in your area. The main point is that you become well-grounded in the theory of one modality, rather than acquiring a smattering of knowledge about several.

- Psychotherapy may seem simple when described or observed. In actual fact, it takes a great deal of subtlety and attention to nuance and the body, and is always grounded in theory. The aim of therapy is not to provide psychobabble explanations to patients. This changes nothing. Do not attempt to do therapy without adequate professional training and supervision.
- Your psychotherapy experience will enhance your comfort level with emotions, and this alone will benefit your patients, since they will now know that it is safe to express them.
- The presenting issue is frequently not the major one. Your role may be to help patients form sharper images of what they really want and need.
- Try to avoid offering advice for psychological problems. It might seem expeditious, but really it mostly addresses the superficial issue and disempowers your patients.
- Anticipate that patients have conflicting emotions, e.g., over treatment options, even if they express only one. Your role is to help the conflicts come to the surface so they can be clearly expressed.
- Frequently all your therapy needs to do is to illuminate problems sufficiently so that your patients recognize the need for formal therapy referral.
- Unexplained fatigue or vague physical symptoms are frequently associated with underlying psychological problems.

References

1   Spagnuolo Lobb M (2003) The theory of self in gestalt therapy. Paper read at the 50th anniversary of the New York Gestalt Institute.

2   Gendlin E (1981) *Focusing*. Bantam, New York.

3   www.focusing.org (accessed 27 June 2005).

4   Weiser Cornell A (1996) *The Power of Focusing. A Practical Guide to Emotional Self-Healing.* New Harbinger Publications, Oakland, CA.

5   Klagsbrun J (2001) Listening and focusing holistic health care tools for nurses. *Nurs Clin North Am.* **36**: 115–30.

6   Perls F (1969) *Ego, Hunger and Aggression.* Random House, New York. (First published in South Africa, 1947.)

7   Perls F, Hefferline R, Goodman P (1951) *Gestalt Therapy: excitement and growth in the human personality.* Julian Press, New York.

8   Greenberg E (1996) When insight hurts: Gestalt therapy and the narcissistically-vulnerable client. *Br Gestalt J.* **5**: 113–20.

18

Conclusion: reclaiming the white coat

> Do not be arrogant because of your knowledge.
> Take counsel with the unlearned as with the learned,
> for the limit of a craft is not fixed
> and there is no craftsman
> whose work is perfect.
>
> The Maxims of Ptah-hotep, 2500 BCE[1]

You have excellent medical skills, your office has a calm and soothing ambience, registration forms are personalized and signal your interest in patients as people, you listen attentively, you are empathetic and supportive, sensitive to issues of shame, trauma, and suffering. You also utilize humor and metaphor appropriately, attend to boundaries and safety, and comfortably form collaborative relationships with your patients and staff. Yes, you are practicing state-of-the-art holistic medicine. All of this, and yet, you still need to do more.

The problem is that you do not work in a vacuum. For many, the healthcare environment is toxic. Around you are practitioners and patients whose autonomy, morale and well-being have been severely impacted by the present healthcare revolution – one which focuses on productivity rather than excellence and ethical practice by external regulation rather than internal. Some entrepreneurial practitioners are thriving, while others are floundering. All the while, medical professional organizations have mostly been frozen into a reactive self-defense mode.

There is also division in the ranks. On the one hand, there are the old guard who protest that 'These young docs don't want to work the hours we did,' and 'They need toughening up; let them learn empathy the hard way.' Then, there are the young Turks demanding 'We want a balanced life,' i.e., limited set hours with a healthy level of leisure time, even though work will most likely become more pressured and even less enjoyable and meaningful in this scenario.

If ever there was a time to recall and reflect upon the history, ethics, and values of the medical profession – and brainstorm creative solutions – it is now. The role of a physician in society used to be a respected and privileged one. Today physicians are pilloried in the courts and often viewed as greedy entrepreneurs. It is time to reclaim medicine as an honorable and noble profession *and to assert leadership*.

The first step is to create a vision. For a glimpse of one, let's turn to a recent newspaper article.

> 'To me it's such a privilege to come to work,' said Mr Robinson, 62. 'The next step is heaven.' Mr Robinson is effusively attentive, greeting each new arrival with a booming voice, a sense of purpose and lavish praise.[2]

Imagine the almost unimaginable that Mr Robinson is Dr Robinson. In fact this quote is from an article in the *New York Times*: 'Standing sentry, armed with towel' in which the professional lives of bathroom (lavatory) attendants are revealed.

It is the rare physician who experiences work as a privilege and greets patients as enthusiastically as Mr Robinson. Many in practice find the odds stacked against them, as one individual reported, 'Just about the time you think you can make both ends meet, somebody moves the ends.'[3]

As I close my eyes to formulate a vision, I imagine the day when passion for medicine flourishes, when time stands still as excitement takes over, and work cannot be distinguished from play; when art is science and science is art; where challenge and skill meet in peak experiences; where process coexists as a value with outcomes; where efficiency and competence set the stage for the physician–patient encounter to be an aesthetic experience; where patients can say, 'Sure it's hard being ill, but my doctors and the staff make all the difference, we are a team.'

Imagine the day when Dr Robinson has as much enthusiasm for his work as Mr Robinson. Utopian for sure, and yet without vision, we cannot create a better future.

There is a glimmer of hope. If those of us who lament on the current state of medicine look back at the past, we can take note that in prior centuries, physicians were limited to healing, and there were few cures. Then science and technology entered the arena, bringing miraculous treatments, yet causing relationship and healing skills to atrophy. While scientific advances were taking place in medicine, less dramatic, but no less significant, advances were occurring in the fields of psychology, psychoneuroimmunology, psychotherapy, and complementary therapies. To date, the medical profession has chosen to remain isolated from these advances to the detriment of patients who intuit the promise of integrative care.

In a new paradigm, medicine can for the first time in history be truly integrated if it weaves together effective treatment and effective healing modalities. Like artist and scientist Leonardo da Vinci whose work represented 'The transcendent unity of science and art, and the expansive cross-semination (of the two) ...',[4] so may medicine be blessed to enter a new renaissance.

This future will require the leadership of physicians to step up to the plate and to set aside self-interest in favor of creating a new professionalism. I am suggesting a call to ARMS! – A Radical Medical Society where dogma is tossed out, white coats are discarded, and a revolution commences. It will be a revolution driven by ethics, quality of care, and a passion for excellence and meaning. Here core values are reclaimed, and our arms extended in partnership to the public and other healthcare professionals to force a serious re-evaluation of the educational system and the healthcare industry. Only then do we reclaim our white coats, this time with a green thread sewn in to remind us of our lineage and tradition as a healing profession.

Change is not only possible, it is inevitable. The direction it takes depends on every physician who leads rather than accedes to exploitation and abuse. In my workshops on spirituality and medicine, we occasionally end with a mantra of empowerment:

It is my choice:
to see an exam room as just a room or realize that room is sacred space
to be called a healthcare provider, or physician and skillful healer
to view the person in my care as patient or miracle of creation
to hear the patient's words as complaint or lament
to regard medical practice as a chore or as holy work
to be isolated or seek community
to be busy all the time or to live a life of conscious rhythms
to see my life as a series of events or part of a hero's journey
to see my work as ultimately meaningless or part of the Great Unfolding.

References

1   Donaldson F (1959) *The Maxims of Ptah-hotep (2500 BCE)*, p. 16. Vantage Press, New York, NY.

2   *New York Times* (2004) Standing sentry, armed with towel. 9 December.

3   McCandless H (1994) A survival kit for physicians. Back to the basics. *Postgrad Med*. **96**: 61–4.

4   Atalay B (2004) *Math and the Mona Lisa: the art and science of Leonardo da Vinci*, p. xvii. Smithsonian Books, Washington, DC.

Index